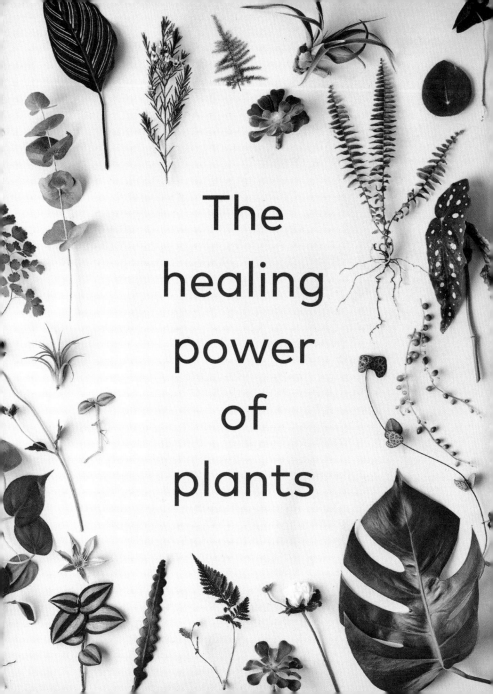

The healing power of plants

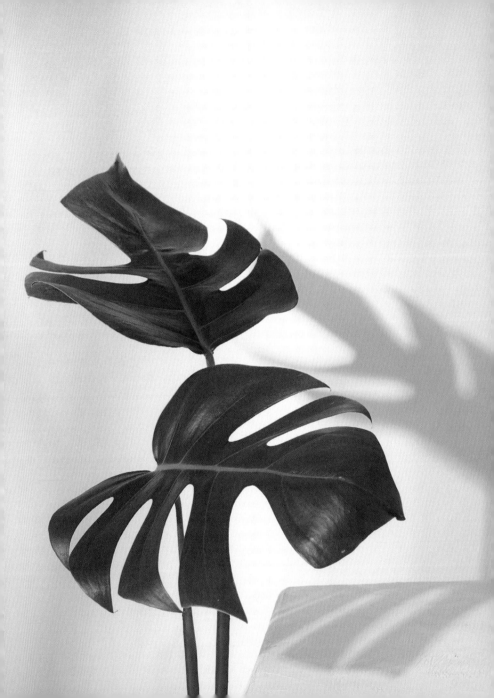

THE HEALING
POWER OF PLANTS

The hero house plants
that will love you back

FRAN BAILEY

POP PRESS

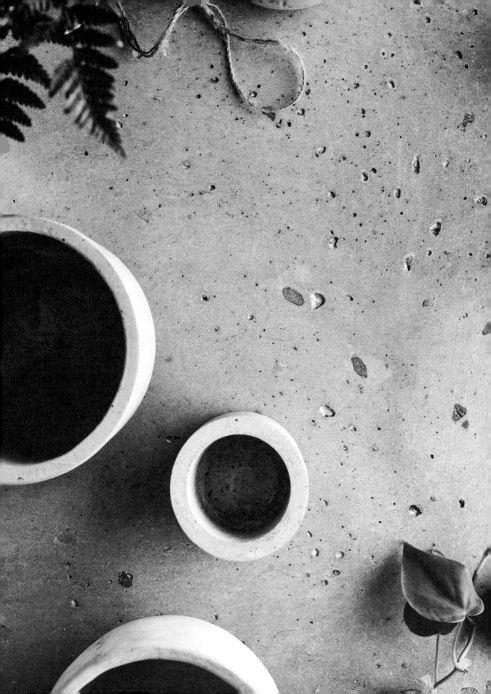

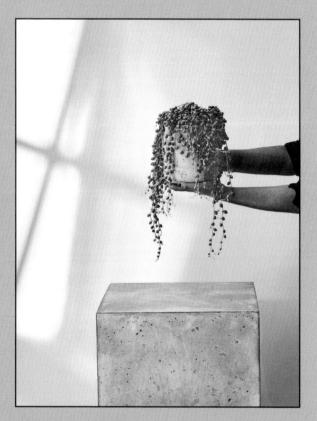

STRING OF PEARLS

Living
with <u>plants</u>

In these modern times, with our ever-growing cities and centrally heated, air-conditioned homes and workplaces, we need plants more than ever. Our connection with plants is primal and we depend on them for our basic human needs, from the air we breathe to the food we eat.

Plants are not only the lungs of the planet, drawing in carbon dioxide and releasing oxygen back into the atmosphere, but also provide us with nourishment, shelter, warmth and medicine. Our ancestors respected plants, utilising the bark, seeds, roots, oils and fruit to maintain good health and combat disease. Their plant knowledge may have been both instinctive and acquired through trial and error, but with each successive generation that wisdom was increased. Today, we have a greater wisdom of the healing power of plants and their extraordinary range of properties: plants can help to keep us alert, calm us when we feel stressed, add goodness to our food and bring joy and beauty to our living and working spaces.

Plants regulate the earth's atmosphere but also work particularly hard for us in our homes. In a bid to clean the air in space stations, scientists at NASA tested and identified the most efficient air-cleaning plants. These tests showed how plants filter out everyday pollutants from the air and release oxygen back into the environment. They add humidity into our dry, centrally heated homes and absorb volatile, often harmful compounds found in furnishings, DIY and cleaning products, and air fresheners.

We also relate to plants in more subtle ways. Although we do not have the same contact with nature our ancestors experienced, we do appear to have an inherent need to be in close proximity to the green world of plants and trees. Walking in the countryside in urban parks, and tending gardens have all been shown to be beneficial for our mental and physical health. But for those of us who live in flats or apartments with no outdoor space, growing and caring for houseplants is a fantastic way of re-establishing our bond with living plants. By bringing plants, such as those from the tropics, into the light and warmth of our home, we invite the outside in and add an exotic feel to our living space.

Caring for our plants can also reduce physiological and psychological stress. Simply looking at and touching plants is thought to lift our mood and when we bring plants into our workspaces, productivity and concentration levels can increase. Even when we are unwell, being in close proximity to plants can also facilitate healing and improve well-being. And plants are also beautiful: they bring a room to life in a way that a sofa or soft furnishings never can. Houseplants are widely available and the choice is huge: there has never been a better time to welcome plants into your home and to learn to care for them, and in turn let them care for you.

HOW TO USE THIS BOOK

This book has been written as a guide to help you learn more about the healing power of plants. Each themed chapter identifies the specific benefits of the plants that are profiled, and even if these are plants that you already have in your home, it is fascinating to learn more about their individual characteristics and needs. The more you know and understand about your plants, the more mutually beneficial your relationship with them will be. Love your plants and they will love you back.

A WORD ABOUT THE NAMING OF PLANTS

The naming of plants is a minefield. As well as the single Latin (botanical) name, most plants have at least a further five or six common names. The plants in this book are identified by one common name as well as the full Latin name (in italics), to avoid the confusion caused by contradictory common names. The Latin name starts with the genus; this is always capitalised and describes the 'group' the plant belongs to. This is followed by the species name, which is always lower case and usually describes a specific characteristic of the individual plant. So in the case of the Panda Plant, Kalanchoe, *tomentosa* means woolly and describes the velvety leaves.

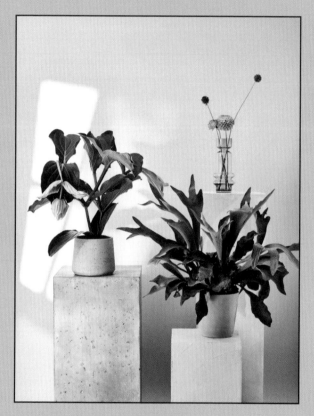

ROSE GRAPE AND STAGHORN FERN

Plants
for <u>calm</u>
and
<u>relaxation</u>

Well-placed plants give a relaxing, restful ambience to any room, and by bringing nature into your home you are helping to create a calmer and more grounded environment. Constantly seeing and being around plants, and even just looking at the colour green, helps us to feel calmer and ready for whatever life throws at us.

PIN-STRIPE CALATHEA
CALATHEA ORNATA

○ **LIGHT** Prefers a shadier position out of bright light, which may scorch the leaves. Look closely and you may notice how the leaves move position to adapt to the light conditions.

〰 **HUMIDITY** Loves high humidity so group Calathea with other plants to create a humid microclimate, or sit the pot in a tray of damp pebbles.

◊ **WATERING** Water thoroughly so the compost is fully soaked and then allow to dry out between watering. If the plant is very thirsty it will roll up its leaves.

✛ **CARE** Calathea is the ideal candidate for brightening up that dingy corner in your living room but will be unhappy if put in a draught. For a healthy plant, feed with half-strength plant food every two weeks throughout the summer season and keep in a warm spot with temperatures above 16°c.

Queen of the forest floor, this extraordinarily beautiful plant really deserves its popularity. This is not a plant for beginners, but given the right conditions it will thrive and can be long-lived. You will also find that the gentle grace of this plant brings a sense of calm to the room. The pink-striped leaves look hand-painted while the deep plum-coloured underside allows the plant to absorb low light. The key to keeping this beauty flourishing is to provide warmth, humidity and filtered light – just as though it were at home in the Amazonian rainforest.

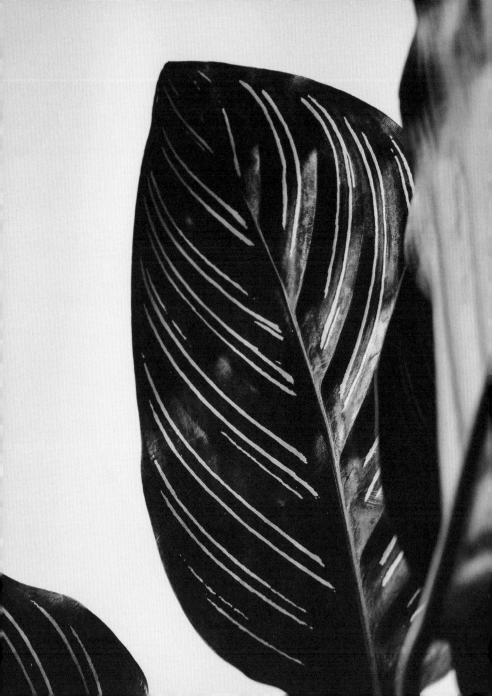

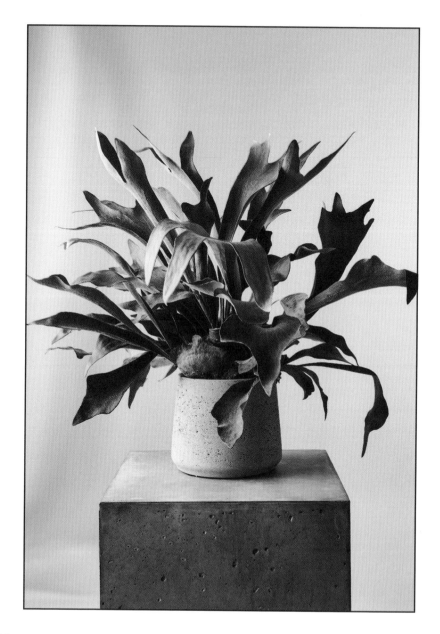

PLANTS FOR CALM AND RELAXATION

STAGHORN FERN
PLATYCERIUM BIFURCATUM

○ **LIGHT** Unlike most other ferns the Staghorn prefers bright but indirect light.

〜 **HUMIDITY** This fern absorbs water through its fronds so responds well to regular misting and high humidity. Mist throughout cooler months, particularly if the central heating is on. A bathroom with sufficient light and ambient humidity is a perfect spot.

◊ **WATERING** Frequency will depend on the heat and humidity levels. Feel behind the low oval-shaped leaves at the base of the plant and if dry submerge the plant in water for a few minutes. Allow compost to dry out between watering – overwatering may rot the plant.

+ **CARE** When repotting, use orchid compost or chipped bark. The smaller, round base fronds turn brown with age: this does not mean that the plant is dying. Any dried shield fronds should not be removed.

The mighty Staghorn is an elegant beast and can make a great houseplant given the right care and attention. The key to success is an understanding of how it grows in its native habitat – the tropics. Like an orchid or air plant, the Staghorn is an epiphyte, attaching itself to the bark of the host tree with its small roots, then absorbing nutrients and water through its green, antler-like fronds. In the wild, the Staghorn can grow to truly epic proportions, cascading from the crook of a tree high up in the forest canopy.

You may have seen these plants mounted on bark pieces – a way of replicating their native forest habitat – and this is the ideal way to grow them at home. They can be grown in pots but their beauty really shines when they are displayed in a hanging basket as a stand-alone specimen. This allows their hanging fronds to cast shadows against the wall, creating a sense of peace and calm.

ASPARAGUS FERN
ASPARAGUS SETACEUS

○ **LIGHT** Prefers bright but indirect light. If the light levels are too low the needles will yellow and drop; too bright and the foliage will scorch.

≈ **HUMIDITY** Enjoys high humidity.

◊ **WATERING** Water regularly during the growing season between spring and autumn; reduce in the winter.

+ **CARE** Keep away from radiators in the winter. When the central heating is on humidity levels may drop, so regular misting will keep your plant happy.

The gentle grace of this plant will aid relaxation when you retreat to the sanctuary of your plant-filled room. Although related to culinary asparagus, it is not edible, nor is it really a fern, so the name of this delicate plant is a little confusing. In the wild this plant is a climber, using the small spines on its stem to scramble up a larger, neighbouring plant. As the fern matures its bushy habit changes, and the feathery fronds become extended and more tendril-like.

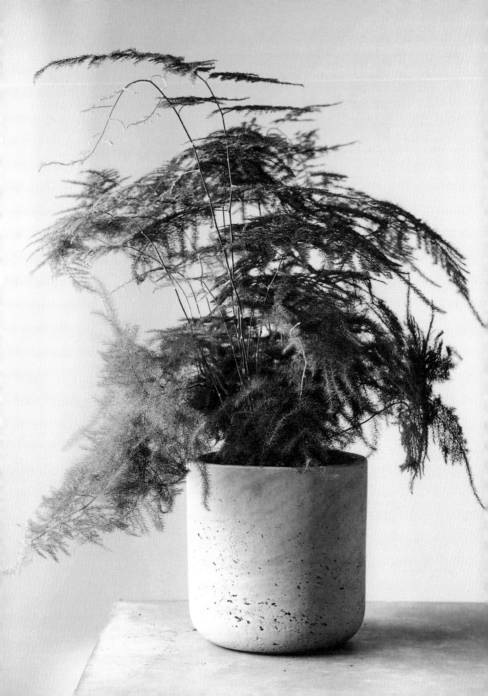

RABBIT-FOOT FERN
PHLEBODIUM AUREUM

○ **LIGHT** Prefers mid- to lower light levels but can tolerate bright indirect light if the temperature remains cool. Direct light will scorch the leaves.

〰 **HUMIDITY** Loves high humidity, so regular misting is beneficial.

◊ **WATERING** Water regularly but moderately: the fern will not tolerate being waterlogged. Make sure excess water can drain away to prevent rotting of the roots and stems.

+ **CARE** Keep your fern away from radiators over the winter and when re-potting use a free-draining medium such as bark chips.

The unusual, soft blue-grey leaves of the Rabbit-foot set it apart from other ferns. Like many other epiphytes, it is found growing on the bark of its host tree in the shaded rainforest canopy. Preferring cool, shady, humid conditions, this is a great plant for a north-facing kitchen or, ideally, a north-facing bathroom that you can fill with ferns to turn it into an oasis of calm and relaxation.

PRAYER PLANT
MARANTA LEUCONERA

○ LIGHT Filtered sunlight.

≋ HUMIDITY Mist regularly
or stand the pot in a tray of
damp pebbles. If the leaf
tips turn brown, this is an
indication that the plant
needs more humidity.

◊ WATERING Keep the
compost moist from spring
to autumn and slightly drier
in winter.

+ CARE Prefers
temperatures above 16ºC
so a warm bathroom is the
ideal spot. Grouping plants
together will create a humid
microclimate that will suit
this plant well.

The leaves fold together at night, like hands
closed in prayer, and open again in the morning
light, giving the plant its common name.
This gentle movement reminds us to take time
out to relax, perhaps spending a few minutes
morning and evening in quiet meditation. For
the detailed veining on the leaves with their
striking dark red undersides, the Prayer Plant
is considered one of the prettiest houseplants.

ROSE GRAPE
MEDINILLA MAGNIFICA

○ **LIGHT** Thrives in bright but indirect light.

〰 **HUMIDITY** Moderate to high. Mist regularly or sit the plant in a tray of damp pebbles.

◊ **WATERING** Allow the compost to dry out fully between watering. When the plant has finished blooming in the winter, reduce watering to around once a fortnight. Increase only when flower stems emerge in the spring.

＋ **CARE** Feed the plant with a high-potash liquid feed every two weeks over the summer months and remove spent flower stems.

A luscious beauty of a plant with arching stems, it has pink bracts and exotic rose-pink flowers. Given the right conditions and a little care, this native of the tropics makes a most impressive houseplant. The Rose Grape loves humid conditions and will really benefit from a daily misting. Focusing on this simple task can help to calm your mind after a hectic day.

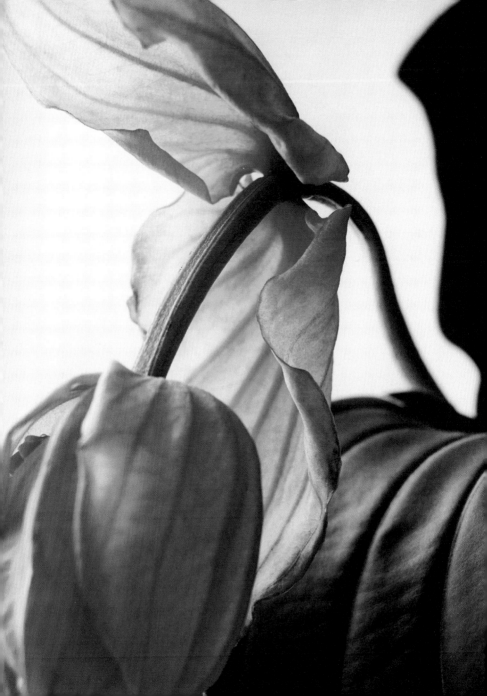

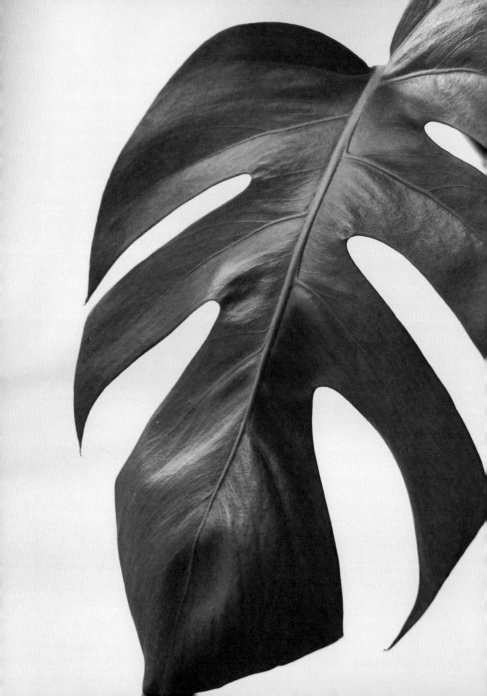

SWISS CHEESE PLANT
MONSTERA DELICIOSA

○ LIGHT Prefers filtered light, out of bright sunlight. Young plants can tolerate a certain amount of shade and will grow well in artificial light. Move into natural light and brighter conditions as the plant matures.

〰 HUMIDITY Moderate humidity; try to mist every few days. If the plant is growing on a moss pole, this can be misted to encourage aerial roots to develop and take hold.

◊ WATERING In the warmer summer months, water only when the top of the compost feels dry. Reduce watering in the winter months.

+ CARE These plants love to climb towards a light source so are ideally placed beneath a skylight or in a stairwell. Aerial roots grow naturally from the stem of the plant: leave or cut off if they get too long. If they are quite low down, push them back into the compost. Wipe the leaves regularly with a damp cloth to remove dust and, if needed, prune in spring.

The easy-to-care-for *Monstera*, a houseplant hero, is so-named because the dark green, heart-shaped leaves of the young plants develop holes as they mature. They are natural climbers and are often sold tied to a mossy pole. A happy Swiss Cheese Plant will grow rapidly and become a floor-standing focal point, its grandeur imbuing the indoor environment with a sense of peace and calm.

AIR PLANTS
TILLANDSIA

○ **LIGHT** Bright light but out of direct sun.

≋ **HUMIDITY** Occasional misting is beneficial to prevent the plants from drying out.

◊ **WATERING** Sit the plants in a shallow tray of tepid water – preferably rainwater or boiled and cooled tap water – once a week for 30 minutes. Remove from the water and let the plants dry fully to avoid the risk of mould or rot.

+ **CARE** Air plants like warmth and good air circulation. Replicate their natural habitat by growing air plants on a piece of natural wood or bark. Never stick the plants on to the wood because the chemicals in adhesives will seriously harm them.

Few plants are easier to care for than these delicate little plants that absorb water and nutrients through their leaves rather than their roots, and therefore need no soil or pot to grow in. They are epiphytes, which do not feed off their host plant but use their roots to anchor themselves to its bark or branches. Most air plants flower annually with surprisingly large and colourful blooms. They will happily sit on a narrow shelf, creating a small area of calm that is ideal for those of us with limited space.

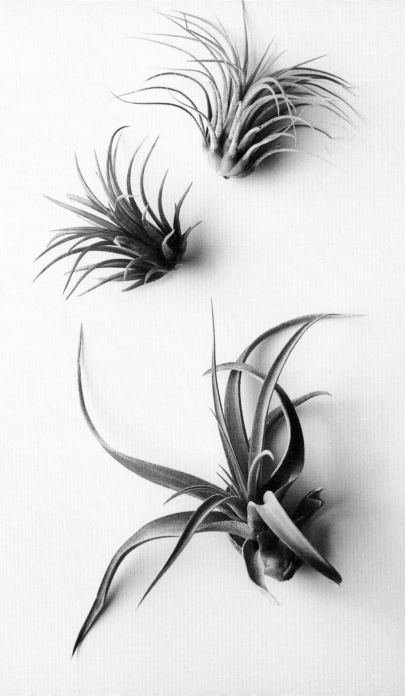

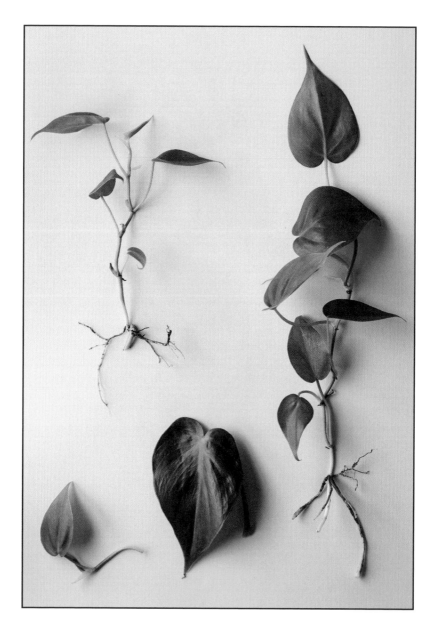

PLANTS FOR CALM AND RELAXATION

HEART LEAF
PHILODENDRON SCANDENS

○ **LIGHT** Prefers filtered light to moderate shade. In hot sun the leaves will scorch and turn yellow.

))) **HUMIDITY** Warm, humid conditions will help this plant to thrive. Mist regularly or sit the plant in a deep saucer of damp pebbles.

◊ **WATERING** Keep the compost moist between spring and autumn; in the winter months water only when the compost feels dry.

+ **CARE** To aid photosynthesis and promote growth, regularly clean dust from the leaves with a damp cloth. To encourage the plant to bush out, pinch out the growing tips. The pruned cuttings will root easily in water (see Propagation p.172).

If you're looking for the 'jungle effect' then this is the plant for you. Fast-growing and easy to care for, it can be placed up high to cascade down a shelving unit or planted low and trained on wires or a mossy pole to scramble upwards. In very modern or minimalist surroundings, the rounded, heart-shaped leaves can soften hard edges and create a green focal point to aid relaxation.

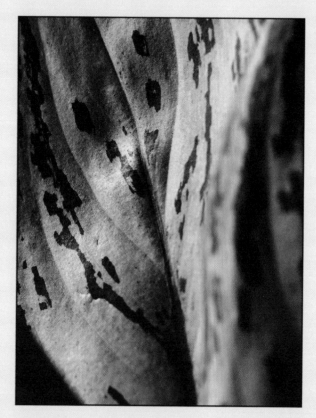

CHINESE EVERGREEN

Plants for a breath of <u>fresh air</u>

The harmful effect of toxins found in pollution in urban areas is well documented, but did you know that the inside of our home may also be polluted? Formaldehyde, benzine and other toxic chemicals are released from soft furnishings, paint, cleaning products and paraffin-based candles; and can lead to respiratory problems and allergies. When NASA needed the most effective air-cleaning plants for their space stations the Snake Plant, Bamboo Palm and the humble ivy came top of the list. On average, we spend more than 90 per cent of our time indoors so it makes sense to reduce harmful toxins by purifying the air in our homes using plants.

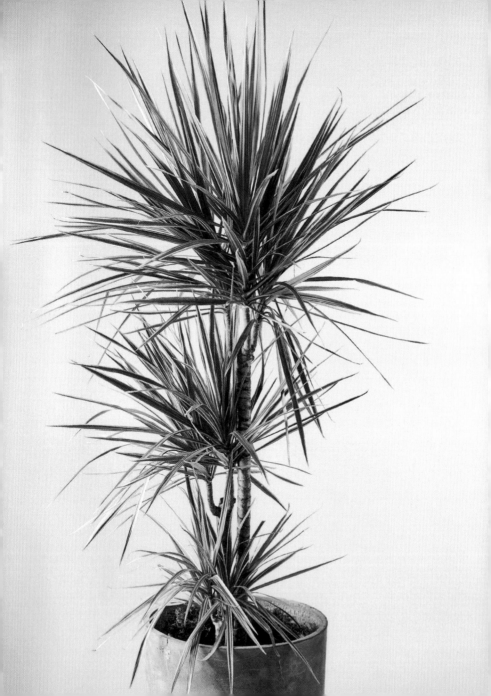

DRAGON PLANT
DRACENA MARGINATA

○ **LIGHT** Filtered sun or light shade. The colour contrast on the leaves will fade if the plant is placed in direct sun.

〰 **HUMIDITY** Moderate. Group with other plants to increase humidity.

◊ **WATERING** Keep the compost moist from spring to autumn and then reduce water in the winter. Will not tolerate being waterlogged.

+ **CARE** To reduce the plant's size, prune back overlong stems or those that spoil the shape. Leaf margins turning brown may be a sign of under- or overwatering, or that the plant is placed in a draught.

This deservedly popular plant likes to stick around – it is both long-lived and easy to care for, potentially growing to a stately height of 3 metres. It is one of the best air purifiers, removing benzene, trichloroethylene and formaldehyde (chemicals that have been linked to cancer and respiratory problems) from indoor air so keep it with you when you move house and it will continue to clean the air as it goes. Clustering this plant with a few others to make a healthy microclimate will also help to increase daytime oxygen in your home.

SPIDER PLANT
CHLOROPHYTUM COMOSUM

○ **LIGHT** Filtered sun or light shade.

))) **HUMIDITY** Low.

◊ **WATERING** Keep the compost moist from spring to autumn and then allow the compost to dry out between watering in the winter. The fleshy, water-holding tuberous roots tolerate a degree of drought.

✛ **CARE** Propagate by cutting plantlets from the parent plant and pot them on individually in small pots.

A staple plant in every household in the 1970s, the Spider Plant is not only one of the easiest houseplants to grow but also the number one air-cleaning plant for beginners. Formaldehyde and xylene, often found in soft furnishings, solvents and adhesives, can build up inside your home causing symptoms such as dizziness, coughing, nausea and headaches, and this popular plant can remove them. Spider Plants look really pretty growing in a basket or a pot in a macramé hanger, from where they send out flowering shoots that eventually grow into baby 'spiders'.

COMMON OR ENGLISH IVY
HEDERA HELIX

○ **LIGHT** Prefers bright but indirect light, but will also tolerate a shady corner.

〰 **HUMIDITY** Moderate.

◊ **WATERING** Keep the compost moist in the summer months but allow the compost to dry out between watering in cooler weather.

✛ **CARE** Larger ivies will need a support such as a frame or canes; small plants can be left to trail down from a high shelf.

Commonly seen trailing over walls in the urban landscape or scrambling up tree trunks in the woods, ivy isn't usually thought of as a houseplant. However, this attractive vine has a very fast growth rate, which makes it an excellent candidate for purifying the air around us. It is not only effective in filtering out formaldehyde and xylene (found in some cleaning products) but also traps airborne particulates such as mould, smoke and dust, which may affect allergy sufferers. There are several varieties of ivy with different leaf shapes, size, colours and patterns.

FLAMINGO FLOWER
ANTHURIUM ANDRAEANUM

○ **LIGHT** Bright, indirect light; avoid direct sunlight.

〰 **HUMIDITY** Moderate, mist often.

◊ **WATERING** Water regularly and do not allow to dry out, but ensure the compost is very free-draining and the base of the pot is not left sitting in water.

✛ **CARE** Add bark chips to the compost to aid drainage. Yellowing leaves may indicate that your plant needs re-potting.

These tropical plants are usually grown for their colourful, waxy spathes but the dark green, arrow-shaped leaves are seriously good-looking, too. Easy to care for and suited to life as a houseplant, Flamingo Flowers like warm and humid conditions in bright but indirect light. NASA lists this as a top plant for filtering ammonia, xylene and formaldehyde from the air.

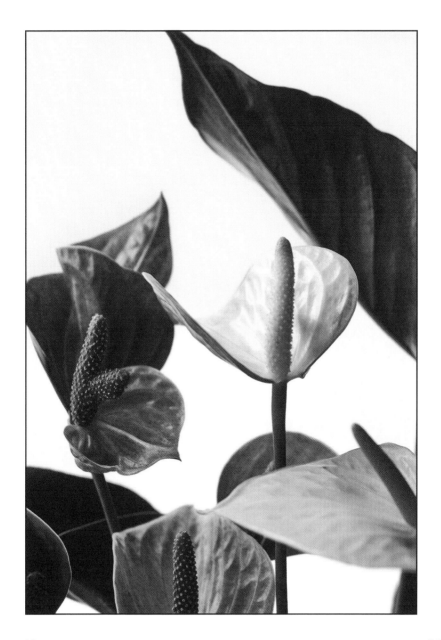

CHINESE EVERGREEN
AGLAONEMA

○ **LIGHT** Prefers low light conditions; keep out of strong sunlight.

≈ **HUMIDITY** Moderate; occasionally spray the leaves with tepid water.

◊ **WATERING** Keep the compost moist during the summer months but reduce water when the light levels drop in winter. Do not allow the pot to stand in water as this may cause root rot.

+ **CARE** Keep the plant out of draughts. All parts of the plant are poisonous if eaten.

A delicate little plant, this evergreen has spear-shaped leaves usually patterned with cream, pink or silver. Perfect for a shady corner in a small flat, it is a slow-growing plant with a maximum height of 50cm. Although small, it has strong air-purifying properties and removes industrial toxins such as formaldehyde and benzene, while increasing daytime oxygen.

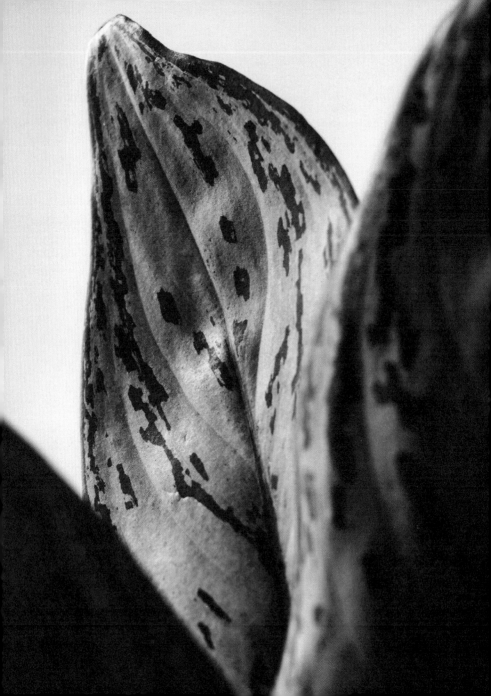

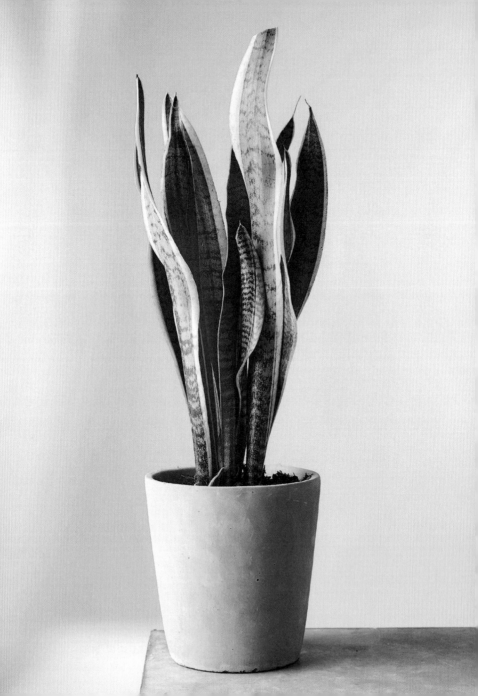

SNAKE PLANT
SANSEVIERIA TRIFASCIATA

○ **LIGHT** Thrives on warmth and light, but tolerates shade well.

≋ **HUMIDITY** Low.

◊ **WATERING** Very sparingly, about once every two weeks and once a month in winter.

✛ **CARE** When the plant outgrows its pot, remove and divide into two smaller plants (see Propagation p.174).

Queen of the air cleaners, this robust plant has been shown in NASA tests to remove benzene, formaldehyde, trichloroethylene and xylene from the air. It also refreshes the indoor environment with life-giving oxygen. If you were to choose just one plant to aid respiratory problems, this is the one to pick. Also known as the 'rough and tough' plant, this *Sansevieria* is virtually bulletproof. It grows slowly, thrives on neglect and will last for years providing you do not overdo the watering.

DEVIL'S IVY
EPIPREMNUM AUREUM

○ **LIGHT** Filtered light or moderate shade.

≋ **HUMIDITY** Moderate

◊ **WATERING** Between spring and autumn allow the compost to dry out between watering. In the winter, keep the compost just moist.

+ **CARE** If growing as a climber, tie the stems into a frame or trellis. Cuttings root easily in water (see Propagation p.172).

This tough little plant is perfect for a beginner – very forgiving if neglected, it can also handle poor light conditions and erratic watering. In its native Polynesia, the vine can grow to 20 metres as it clambers up into the forest canopy. Thankfully, it will grow at a far more moderate pace in the confines of a pot and you can always keep it in check with regular pruning. Display it up high on a shelf where the glossy yellow and green leaves can cascade elegantly to the floor, while also filtering benzene, formaldehyde and xylene from the air.

PARLOUR PALM
CHAMAEDOREA ELEGANS

○ **LIGHT** Dappled shade.

〰 **HUMIDITY** Moderate to high; likes regular misting. Ideally place in a kitchen or bathroom.

◊ **WATERING** In the summer months allow the top of the compost to dry out between watering and water only very sparingly in the winter. Palms do not like to be overwatered.

✛ **CARE** Fronds will naturally turn brown at the base of the palm and can be cut off. If the tips of the leaves turn brown, the air may be too dry or there may be a draught.

Popular since Victorian times, this elegant palm has lush, feathery foliage. Like other indoor palms, it can help to give your space a touch of the tropical oasis. As well as being highly effective in removing formaldehyde, this palm is also very easy to grow and can reach over 3 metres, creating a pleasing focal point. To maintain a happy plant, keep it away from radiators or other direct sources of heat.

PEACE LILY
SPATHIPHYLLUM

○ **LIGHT** Filtered sun or
light shade.

⌇ **HUMIDITY** Moderate.

◊ **WATERING** Allow the
compost to dry out between
watering but do not allow
the plant to wilt; this will
cause the deep green leaves
to loose their sheen and
start to turn yellow.

+ **CARE** Easy. Over time
the white spadix (flower
spike) will fade to green
and eventually turn brown.
At this point, remove it
from the plant.

An unassuming but rewarding plant, the Peace
Lily will bloom reliably for many months,
withstanding poor light levels as well as a degree
of neglect. At the same time it will work hard
to remove volatile organic compounds, such as
solvents, from the atmosphere. Tests have also
shown that the plant is capable of removing
airborne mould, which can alleviate allergy and
asthma symptoms. As an added bonus, the Peace
Lily may help you get a good night's sleep.

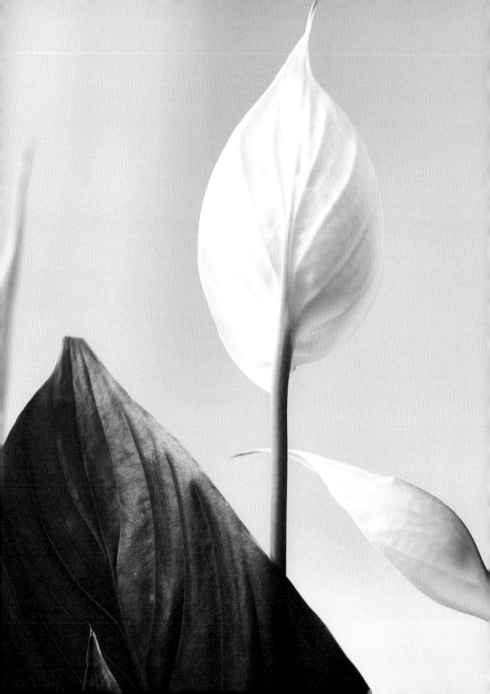

BOSTON FERN
NEPHROLEPIS EXALTATA

○ **LIGHT** Filtered sun or light shade.

〰 **HUMIDITY** Moderate to high; mist your plant regularly.

◊ **WATERING** Between spring and autumn keep the compost just moist, allowing it to dry out between watering in the winter months.

+ **CARE** Moderately easy. If the frond tips turn brown, this may be a sign that the plant has dried out and needs higher humidity. To keep it looking good, cut back any scorched leaf fronds to the base. A fortnightly liquid feed throughout the warmer months is beneficial.

This elegant fern is a cool customer, preferring light shade and humid conditions. It will feel most at home in your bathroom. Given the right conditions, it will grow into a magnificent creature 1 metre in diameter and will look its best displayed in a hanging basket or macramé hanger. In dry interiors, especially during the winter months when the central heating is on, create the humidity your fern needs by setting it on a tray of damp pebbles. In turn, the fern will remove formaldehyde and xylene and ease symptoms associated with these pollutants, such as headaches and respiratory ailments.

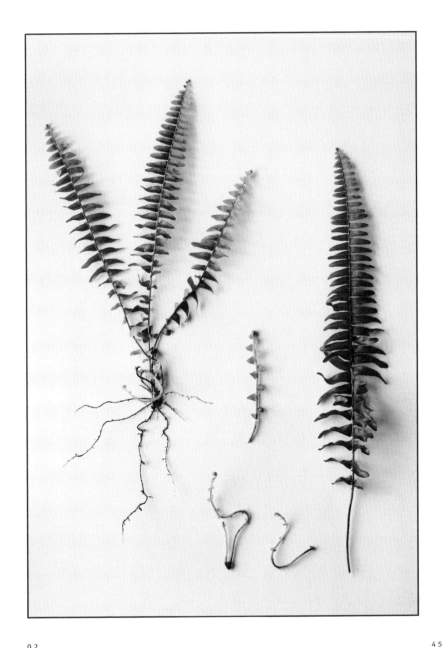

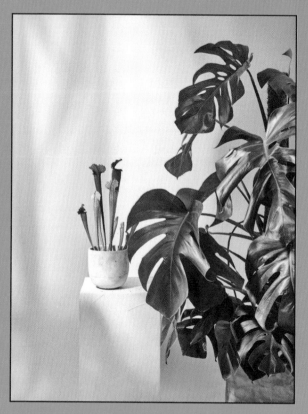

PITCHER PLANT AND SWISS CHEESE PLANT

Plants that generate an abundance of oxygen can have a calming effect, reducing insomnia. Through a process of photosynthesis known as CAM (crassulacean acid metabolism), some release oxygen at night rather than through the day. Other plants filter pollutants, as well as airborne microbes such as mould spores and bacteria. These can infect your airways and disturb sleep patterns. Some houseplants can also lower blood pressure, reduce heart rate and soothe your senses.

Plants

for a

good night's

sleep

LAVENDER
LAVANDULA

○ **LIGHT** Keep in a bright spot beside the window.

≋ **HUMIDITY** Low.

◊ **WATERING** Soak the compost and allow to dry out before repeat watering.

✛ **CARE** When the flowers have died back, put the plant in a frost-proof pot to overwinter outside, then bring it back inside when it blooms again.

For those who find it hard to unwind, Lavender (opposite) can aid relaxation. The calming scent of lavender is known to lower blood pressure and reduce the heart rate, which in turn will decrease stress levels to aid a good night's sleep. Essential oil of lavender is commonly used as a room or pillow spray and the flowers have the same calming benefits, while at the same time adding beauty and scent to your bedroom.

SCENTED JASMINE
JASMINUM POLYANTHUM

○ **LIGHT** Filtered sun, out of direct light.

≋ **HUMIDITY** Low.

◊ **WATERING** Do not let the plant dry out when in flower or the blooms will turn brown and drop prematurely.

✛ **CARE** Apply a liquid fertilizer every two weeks between spring and summer.

Filling your bedroom with its heady perfume, this beautiful flowering climber will soothe your senses and lull you to sleep. It is normally sold growing on a hoop or wrapped around a pyramid frame and brightens up the dark days of midwinter, when it flowers. Once blooming is over and temperatures rise, put the plant outside.

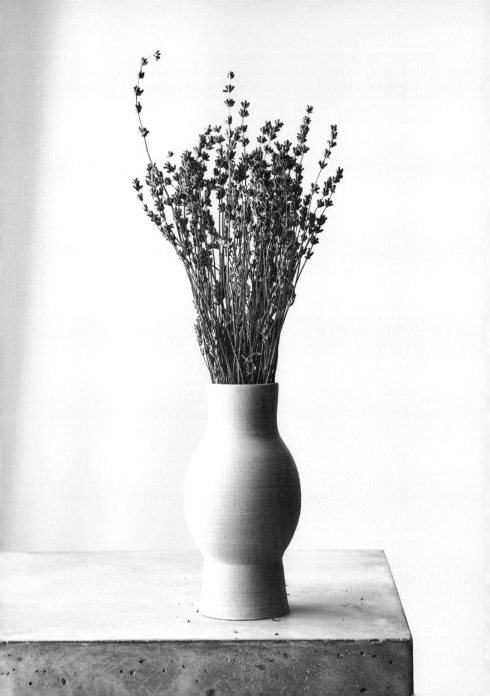

ARECA PALM
DYPSIS LUTESCENS

○ **LIGHT** Prefers filtered sunlight.

〰 **HUMIDITY** Moderate; mist every few days or stand on a tray of damp pebbles.

◊ **WATERING** Over the warmer summer months water well, especially if placed in a brighter spot. Reduce the frequency of watering over the winter.

✛ **CARE** The size of the pot will determine the size of your palm so if you want to restrict its growth, keep it in a smaller pot. This palm should need re-potting only every five to ten years.

One of the easiest palms to grow as a houseplant, the Areca can grow up to 2 metres and will make a great focal point in your bedroom if you're lucky enough to have the space. There are three main benefits to growing this plant. Firstly it is a natural humidifier and a large plant may transpire up to a litre of moisture a day! Secondly, it cleanses the air of harmful toxins, including formaldehyde, which can irritate the skin. Finally, this heroic plant emits oxygen at night and is one of the very best at promoting restful sleep.

GARDENIA

GARDENIA JASMINOIDES

○ LIGHT Filtered light.

≋ HUMIDITY High; mist the leaves (but not the flowers) regularly or stand on a tray of pebbles and water.

◊ WATERING Keep the compost moist. If possible, use rainwater, boiled and cooled tap water or distilled water. Reduce water in winter.

+ CARE Keep in a warm room well out of draughts. Cold, dry conditions may cause the flower buds to drop.

Gardenias can be tricky to grow, but they are oh so beautiful. The perfume is, literally, intoxicating and in tests the scent, which induced an extremely deep and restful night's sleep, was as effective as sleeping tablets and valium. Invest a little time into the care of this plant and you will be richly rewarded.

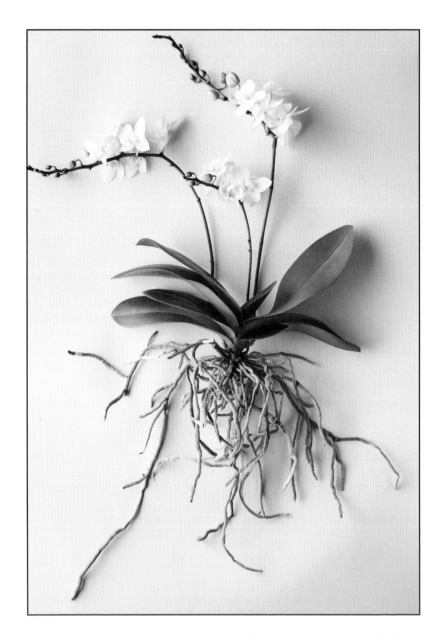

PLANTS FOR A GOOD NIGHT'S SLEEP

MOTH ORCHID
PHALAENOPSIS

○ **LIGHT** Prefers bright but filtered light.

〰 **HUMIDITY** Moderate; will enjoy occasional misting.

◊ **WATERING** Orchids do not require compost and are most commonly grown in chipped bark or specialist orchid compost. They hate to be waterlogged. The aerial roots, however, prefer not to dry out so give your plant a regular soaking and ensure all the water drains through the pot. If possible use rainwater, distilled or boiled and cooled water.

✛ **CARE** The plant can bloom at any time of the year. To encourage a new flush, cut the faded flower stem just above the second horizontal band on the stem.

These popular orchids with their exotic blooms have become so widely available, often looking a little sad in their plastic wrappers at the supermarket checkout, that we've perhaps started to take them for granted. Group with other rainforest natives such as Calathea (see p.12) or among ferns with dark foliage that will act as a foil for the pretty moth orchid, allowing its beauty to shine out. A perfect plant for the bedroom, the Moth Orchid emits health-giving oxygen at night and banishes xylene, a toxin found in some paints and varnishes.

MONEY TREE
PACHIRA AQUATICA

○ **LIGHT** Bright but indirect light.

♒ **HUMIDITY** Enjoys high humidity so mist every few days or stand in a tray of damp pebbles.

◊ **WATERING** Water weekly from spring to autumn or when the top of the compost is dry. Reduce watering in winter.

✛ **CARE** Keep the plant bushy and compact by pinching out the stem tips. As with some other houseplants, the Money Tree does not like changes of scene. When you buy a new plant it may shed a few leaves. Just give it a little time to settle into its new home.

Said to bring good luck and fortune, the Money Tree is considered auspicious in Asia where it is employed by practitioners of feng shui. Growing wild in the swamps of its native South America, the tree can reach a height of 18 metres, but a small pot and careful pruning will keep it compact and suitable as a houseplant. The soft stems of the young plant are quite malleable and are often sold braided, hence the other common name, Plaited Plant. Easy to care for and very decorative, the Money Tree has air-cleaning properties and is a great plant to have in your bedroom if you suffer from respiratory problems at night.

CHRISTMAS CACTUS
SCHLUMBERGERA TRUNCATA

○ LIGHT Dappled,
indirect light.

〰 HUMIDITY Moderate;
will benefit from
regular misting.

◊ WATERING Keep the
compost moist but never
soak or leave the plant to
sit in water; it hates to have
wet feet. Use rainwater
if possible.

+ CARE After flowering
your cactus requires a rest
period, so cut back on
watering and feeding for
the next few months and
keep in a cool but frost-free
place. In the spring, bring
back into the warmth
and light and water more
regularly. You will soon
notice small flower
buds appearing.

This pretty forest cactus flowers in the winter, hence its name. It is easy to grow and with a little care and attention can be encouraged to bloom just in time for Christmas. As well as looking pretty in your bedroom over the festive period, it will work hard to improve the quality of the air by emitting oxygen while you sleep. Like other clean-air heroes, it removes airborne toxins including formaldehyde and benzene.

PITCHER PLANT
SARRACENIA

○ **LIGHT** Bright sun.

〣 **HUMIDITY** High humidity.

◊ **WATERING** Carnivorous plants are bog-dwellers and prefer continuously moist but free-draining compost.

✛ **CARE** For best results they should be planted in a 50/50 mix of sphagnum moss and coarse sand. Carnivorous plants prefer cool conditions in the winter months when they will become semi-dormant. Water with rainwater or distilled water as the chemicals in tap water will harm them. Protect your plants from hot, dry air and draughts.

Is there anything more stressful than lying in bed on a warm summer's night listening to the high-pitched whine of a bloodthirsty mosquito? Numbers are on the increase now our summers seem to be getting warmer and these troublesome insects are active from dusk to dawn. Carnivorous plants may help to control these pests without the need for chemical sprays. There are three different groups of carnivorous plant: the Venus Fly Trap *(Dionaea muscipula)* snaps its fearsome jaws shut when an unlucky fly lands on it; Pitcher Plants *(Sarracenia)* drown their prey in leaf tubes filled with digestive juices; and insects cannot escape from the sticky leaf pads of Sundews *(Drosera)*. Group a collection of carnivorous plants in your bedroom for peace and quiet, letting them do their work while you get a peaceful night's sleep.

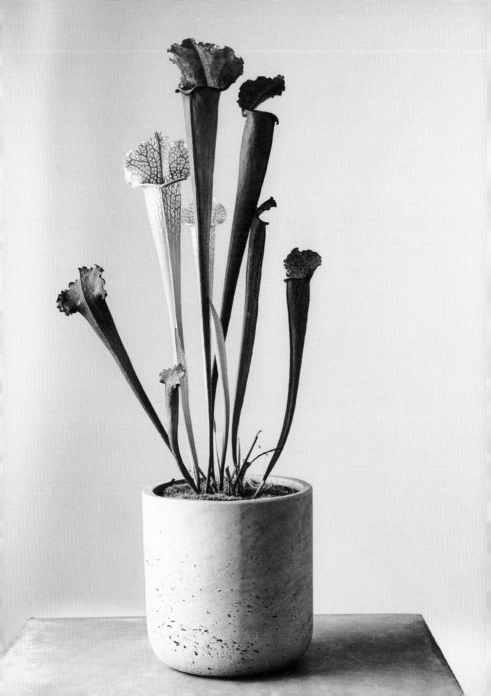

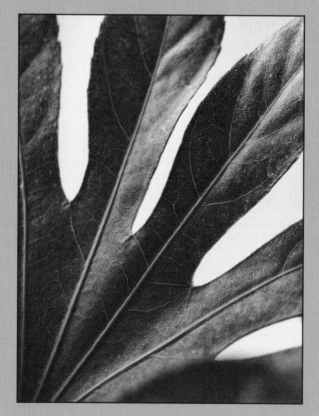

FATSIA

Just being in the presence of plants can instantly relax you and lighten your mood, improving both mental and physical well-being. Transforming your environment into a more positive space with houseplants also helps increase feelings of comfort, security and safety. Caring for your plants reminds you to take more care of yourself.

Plants
to improve
well-being

VELVET PLANT
GYNURA AURANTIACA

○ **LIGHT** Bright but indirect light is ideal; the purple colour will fade if conditions are not bright enough.

〰 **HUMIDITY** Low; the leaves prefer not to be misted.

◊ **WATERING** Take care not to overwater this plant as it is susceptible to root rot. Make sure that the top 2cm of the compost is dry before watering.

✛ **CARE** The plant can become leggy. Encourage bushy growth by pinching out the growing tips.

Unusual and very distinctive, this gothic-looking plant has deep green leaves covered in soft purple hairs, making it velvety to the touch. Physical interaction with our plants, such as touching the leaves, can reduce stress levels and increase our psychological well-being. And it's mutually beneficial: touching the leaves causes biochemical changes to occur within the plant, boosting its defences against pests and diseases and encouraging stronger stem growth.

The Velvet Plant is quite short-lived, perhaps lasting just two or three years as a houseplant. It is, however, very fast growing and easy to propagate by stem cuttings, so in theory the mother plant can provide offspring for years to come.

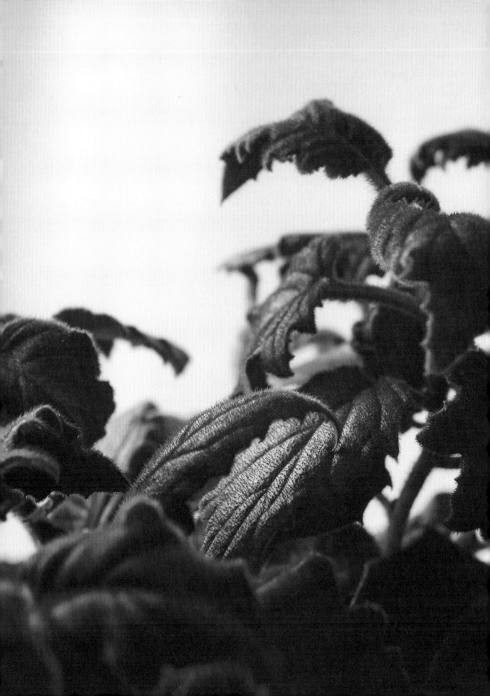

'ATTAR OF ROSES'
SCENTED GERANIUM
PELARGONIUM

○ **LIGHT** Geraniums are sun-worshippers so keep on a sunny windowsill.

〰 **HUMIDITY** Low.

◊ **WATERING** Water only when the soil has completely dried out.

✛ **CARE** Keep away from direct sources of heat, such as open fires and radiators, in the cooler months. Plants can also be kept in a frost-free porch over winter. To boost growth in the spring, set on a sunny windowsill and feed with a general fertilizer. The leaves can be infused in hot water to make a soothing, rose-flavoured tea.

Harsh, synthetic room fragrances, such as sprays, plug-ins and scented candles, are a sure way to pollute your home with headache-inducing chemicals. But why have artificial scent when you can have the real thing? In a bid to attract pollinators, most plants emit fragrance via their flowers, but it is the leaves of the rose geranium that contain the valuable essential oils. When rubbed between your fingers, they will release a burst of mood-boosting scent.

SAGO PALM
CYCAS REVOLUTA

○ LIGHT Bright but
indirect light.

≈ HUMIDITY Moderate;
mist the leaves in summer.

◊ WATERING In the summer
months, water only once the
compost has dried out. Keep
it virtually dry in the winter.

+ CARE Take care not to
overwater and avoid
watering the crown, which
may cause rot. All parts
of the plant are toxic.

These ancient plants have been around since
the era of the dinosaurs and although they look
like palms they are cycads – primitive, fern-like
evergreens. They are easy to care for and very
slow growing, so you may have this beautiful
plant for life. Be sure to take it with you when
you move house because it's a perfect stress-
buster, working hard to purify the air, remove
toxins and add moisture to the atmosphere.

FATSIA

FATSIA JAPONICA

○ LIGHT Prefers filtered
sun or light shade.

≋ HUMIDITY Low
to moderate.

◊ WATERING From spring
to autumn give the plant
a good soak when the
compost feels dry. Reduce
water in the cooler months.
The leaves will droop
dramatically if the plant has
been left to dry out and if
this happens, submerge the
whole pot in a bucket full of
water for 10 minutes, then
remove and allow to drain
completely. Fatsia is very
forgiving and will soon
come back to life.

+ CARE Keep in a cool spot
over the winter, away from
any direct sources of heat,
such as fireplace or radiator.

A great choice for novice growers, this
architectural plant has big, glossy green leaves
that look like hands. Alone, it makes a good
statement plant, but if grouped with other
large-leaved tropical plants, the microclimate
they create will humidify your room. Balanced
humidity indoors is vital for your well-being,
especially in the winter months when central
heating can dry out the air, as well as the nose
and throat, and increase the chance of catching
a cold or respiratory problems. Increasing the
humidity levels by introducing this handsome
plant will naturally ease discomfort.

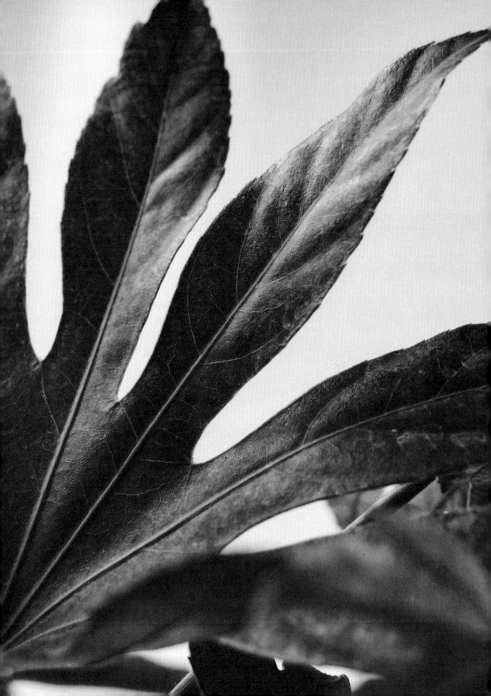

FURRY FEATHER
CALATHEA RUFIBARBA

○ **LIGHT** Direct, diffused light; leaves will easily scorch if placed in direct sun.

∿ **HUMIDITY** High; stand the pot on a tray of damp pebbles and mist the leaves regularly.

◊ **WATERING** Keep the compost moist during the warmer months and then reduce in the winter. Leaf curling is a sure sign that the plant is thirsty.

+ **CARE** Wipe the leaves clean with a damp cloth to remove dust build-up. Never use commercial leaf shine as this will damage the delicate leaves.

Another beauty from the *Calathea* group of plants, this one also has striking tropical foliage and deserves a place in your home. The Furry Feather is especially popular because the leaves, with undersides in a deep shade of burgundy, are covered in tiny hairs, making them soft and velvety to the touch. Making contact with plants by simply stroking their leaves and stems has been shown to improve our mental well-being, making us feel calmer and happier.

MOSS GARDEN

— Clear glass container with a wide neck and a lid
— Moss, decorative pebbles, stones and pieces of foraged wood
— Potting compost, fine gravel and activated charcoal

+ CARE Keep the moss garden out of bright sunlight, opening the lid of the container and misting the moss a few times a week; it should not be allowed to dry out. Sealing the container reduces evaporation and creates a mini-, self-sustaining microclimate. But if you cannot see condensation on the glass then the atmosphere is too dry and the mosses will need additional moisture.

The benefits of indoor gardening for our mental well-being are considered to be on a par with getting our hands dirty down at the allotment – which is great news for the 80 per cent of us who are urban dwellers and may not have access to a garden. Making a table-top moss garden in a terrarium or large glass jar is a great way of bringing the outdoors in. Using just stones, wood and living moss, you can recreate a beautiful miniature forest in your home.

HOW TO

Pour a layer of fine gravel into the base of the jar. Add a layer of potting compost to which you have added two teaspoons of activated charcoal to prevent the growth of fungi. Place the moss onto the compost and carefully arrange a few decorative stones and pieces of wood on top (using tongs if necessary). Mist the moss and seal the container.

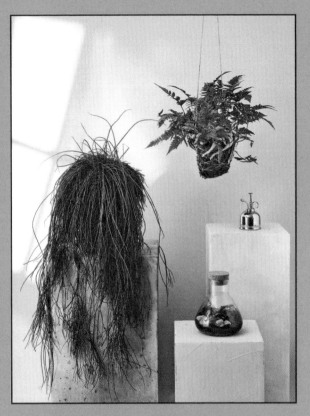

MISTLETOE CACTUS, KOKEDAMA FERN
AND TERRARIUM

CHAPTER 05

Plants

to <u>reduce</u>

<u>stress</u>

According to one of America's foremost
biologists, humans have an innate desire to be
connected with nature and he coined the term
'biophilia' to describe it. Most of us spend large
amounts of time inside artificially lit buildings
and have very little contact with the natural
environment, which can increase feelings of
anxiety and stress. Yet the soil our plants grow in
contains microbes, dubbed 'outdoorphins', these
work as natural anti-depressants, stimulating the
'happiness chemical', serotonin, in our brains.

HOLY BASIL
OCIMUM TENUIFLORUM

○ **LIGHT** Bright sunlit spot.

〰 **HUMIDITY** Moderate.

◊ **WATERING** Let compost dry out between watering then give the plant a good soak.

✛ **CARE** Basil seeds germinate quickly indoors so you can grow a succession of plants all year round.

Known in Ayurvedic medicine as *tulsi*, this herb is a sacred Hindu plant and a tonic for body, mind and spirit. The flowers and leaves emit a characteristic aroma that is known to soothe nerves and reduce anxiety. As a houseplant Holy Basil is also considered a super oxygenator, emitting oxygen for about 20 hours a day. As with all herbs that are grown indoors, it should be kept on a sunny windowsill and away from direct sources of heat in the winter.

WAX FLOWER
HOYA CARNOSA

○ **LIGHT** Bright indirect light.

〰 **HUMIDITY** Moderate; enjoys regular misting.

◊ **WATERING** Keep moist in spring and summer. In winter dry out between watering. Don't let the pot sit in water or roots may rot.

✛ **CARE** Plant in free-draining compost, with bark chips. The plant flowers on the previous year's stems so do not cut these back.

Fill your room with the sweet scent of the delicate Wax Flower for an instant mood boost. The fragrance of the pretty, star-shaped flowers is similar to jasmine with a touch of vanilla and a hint of coconut. Look closely at your plant and you may see a drop of nectar suspended from each flower. If you like a sugar hit in the mornings, go ahead and taste – it's sweet and delicious.

ZEN SAND GARDEN

— a compact plant with a
  symmetrical leaf pattern,
  such as an *Echeveria*
— shallow glass bowl, at least
  three times the diameter of
  your plant
— fine sand and a mini-rake

+ CARE Keep the bowl in
  a bright spot out of direct
  sunlight and water the
  succulent only when the
  sand feels very dry.

In the Japanese Buddhist tradition, creating and tending to Zen gardens is a form of meditation. The act of raking concentric patterns in the sand calms your mind and increases concentration. Focusing on the slow rhythm of the task in hand helps you to let go of stressful thoughts. The technique, called *samon*, serves aesthetic as well as meditative purposes and although it may seem easy, the art of making continuous patterns requires patience and extreme concentration.

HOW TO

Place the plant in one corner of the bowl and fill in all around it with the sand until it is almost level with the top of the bowl but doesn't cover the lower leaves of the plant. Use the rake to make concentric patterns in the sand, adding a few drops of your favourite essential oil to aid concentration whilst raking.

TERRARIUM

— sealed glass bottle or jar
— fine gravel, activated charcoal, multi-purpose compost
— selection of foliage plants and mosses

+ CARE Keep in bright but indirect sunlight and make sure the glass is kept clean so there is enough light for photosynthesis. Some plants will inevitably do better than others: if a small plant dies in the first week, open the lid and carefully remove it, trying not to disturb the others.

A complete ecosystem in a bottle or jar, this beautiful mini-landscape is very easy to plant. And once established, a terrarium is self-sustaining, making it maintenance- and stress-free. You can use any glass jar with a seal, such as a preserving jar – preferably one with a wide neck, which will be a lot easier to work with. Start small and move onto larger vessels as you gain confidence. Small plants that work well in this environment are ferns, mosses and those with striking foliage, such as *Calathea* and *Fittonia*.

HOW TO

Pour a layer of gravel into the base of the jar to a depth of about 5cm and mix in one teaspoon of activated charcoal to prevent fungal growth. Now add a 15cm deep layer of compost. Using your fingers (or a dibber if the neck of the jar is very narrow), make a hole in the compost of a suitable size for the first plant. Remove the plant from its pot, loosen the roots to encourage growth and gently place the plant in the hole, firming the compost around its base. Repeat with the remaining plants, making sure there is space between the plants to allow for growth and air-flow. Once all the plants are firmed in, water the compost so that is wet but not saturated. Leave the lid open for a few days while the plants settle in, water again if the compost looks dry, then seal the lid.

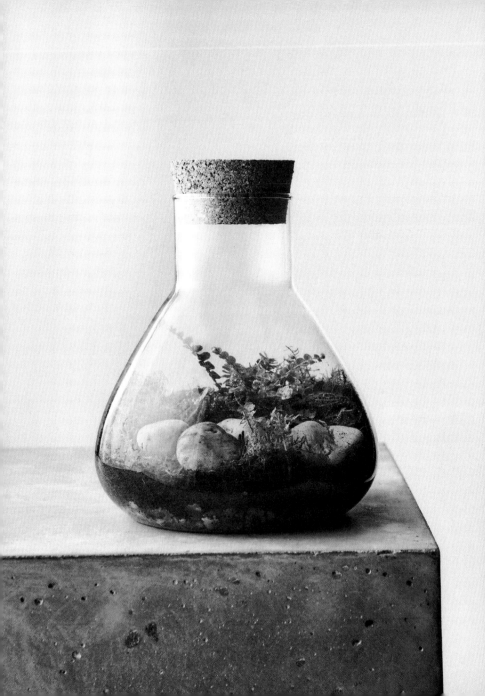

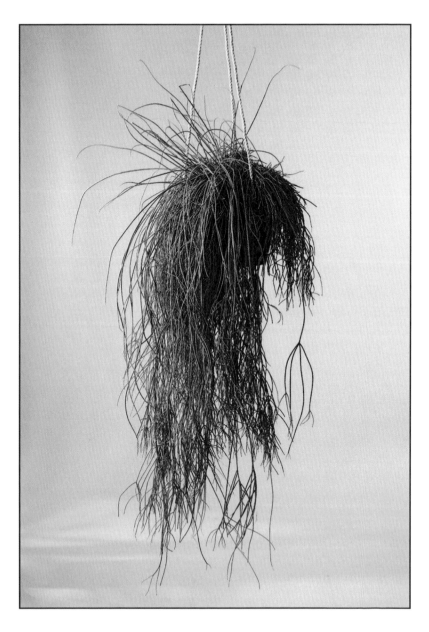

PLANTS TO REDUCE STRESS

MISTLETOE CACTUS
RHIPSALIS BACCIFERA

○ **LIGHT** Indirect, diffused light.

≋ **HUMIDITY** High; enjoys regular misting. As a special treat, give your plant a shower.

◊ **WATERING** Water freely in the summer months, but make sure the pot's drainage holes are clear and the roots are not sitting in water. Ease up a little in the winter months. The stems will shrivel if there is too little moisture.

+ **CARE** Prefers morning sun and shade in the afternoon; the leaves may burn if exposed to strong sunlight. The small white flowers are followed by mistletoe-like white berries.

Minimise the stress in your life by choosing this unusual and beautiful easy-care hanging plant. This cactus, which has no spines, is an epiphyte that grows high up in the rainforest canopy. Unlike desert cacti, this one loves humidity and possesses succulent, water-holding stems. Perfectly suited to life in the bathroom, the Mistletoe Cactus offers something lovely to gaze at while you enjoy a relaxing soak.

KOKEDAMA FERN

WHAT YOU WILL NEED

— ferns
— akadama bonsai soil
— carpet moss
— garden twine

+ **CARE** When the moss
  ball feels light, this is an
  indication the plant needs
  water. Submerge the moss
  ball for 10 to 15 minutes until
  completely saturated, allow
  to drain, then re-position
  your fern in a humid spot
  out of direct sunlight.

The art of Kokedama has its origins in Japan. In
this form of bonsai, a plant is removed from its
pot and the roots are then enveloped first in soil,
then moss, and wrapped with twine to form a ball.
A single plant can be suspended to form a focal
point, or a few can be grouped for more impact,
creating a 'string garden'. You can also sit the plant
in a saucer. Making your own Kokedama at home,
using ferns that flourish in clay soil, is a simple
way to relieve stress. The focus needed to create
such a delicate and beautiful living work of art is
itself a kind of meditation.

HOW TO

Remove the fern from its pot and after gently
shaking loose most of the compost, encase the
roots in a layer of wet akadama soil. Aim to
create a ball of approximately the same volume as
the original pot. Envelop the root ball in carpet
moss and wrap the twine around it to secure the
moss in place.

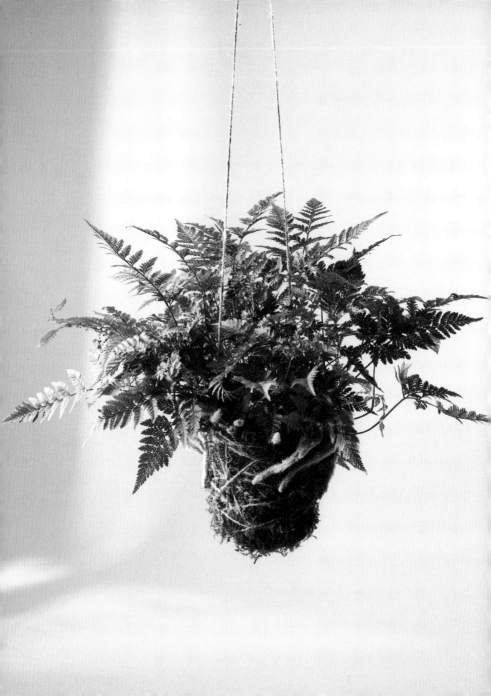

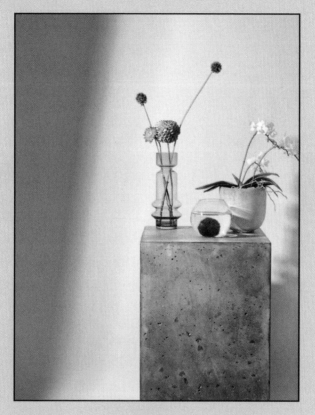

MARIMO WATER GARDEN AND MOTH ORCHID

The simple daily ritual of caring for your plants and watching them thrive can bring happiness and contentment. Tending your plants is a slow, meditative and even humbling experience. Indoor gardening teaches you patience – plants can't be rushed – and also to have hope in the future. Time given over to the care of your plants is repaid when you experience the joy of watching a new leaf unfurl or a small cutting take root. And scientific research confirms that gardening can lift our mood, making us feel happier and more optimistic.

Plants that bring joy and happiness

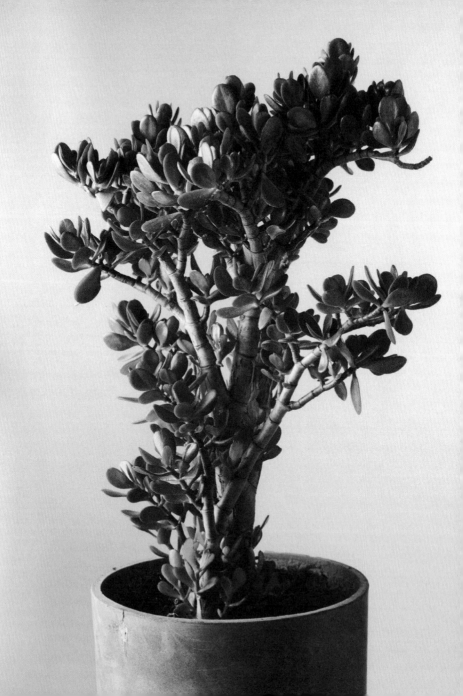

JADE PLANT
CRASSULA OVATA

○ **LIGHT** Bright or indirect light.

〰 **HUMIDITY** Low.

◊ **WATERING** In the summer months, water only when the compost has dried out. In the winter water sparingly – just enough to prevent the leaves from shrivelling up.

✛ **CARE** Re-pot every two to three years. Mature plants can reach a stately 1 metre in height and will make a beautiful feature in any room.

Jade plants are remarkably easy plants to care for, which goes some way to account for their enduring popularity worldwide. They are succulents that hold water in the leaves and stems and prefer to be kept quite dry, even tolerating a certain amount of neglect. In Asian cultures they are associated with good luck, wealth and prosperity: followers of feng shui place them in a southeast corner, where each new leaf growth is said to increase wealth. Although wealth does not equal happiness, with a little investment in the care of this plant you are sure to reap rewards.

STRING OF PEARLS
SENECIO ROWLEYANUS

○ **LIGHT** Bright, indirect light.

〰 **HUMIDITY** Low.

💧 **WATERING** Moderate.
Allow the top of the compost
to dry out between watering
and keep just moist in the
winter to prevent the leaves
from withering.

+ **CARE** The stems root easily
if laid on compost and this is
a great way to increase your
stock or to thicken up your
plant if it's getting a little
thin on top.

In the houseplant popularity stakes, this pretty
little succulent is a winner; and it is a most
joyful-looking plant. Hailing from South Africa,
it has spherical leaves the shape and size of small
peas that have adapted to minimise water loss
while maximising photosynthesis. Look closely
at the bead-like leaves and you will see a dark
green band, a bit like a cat's eye. Known as an
epidermal window, it allows light to enter the
interior of the leaf to increase the surface area
available for photosynthesis. Attractive, clever,
and easy to care for, this plant is the perfect
house guest.

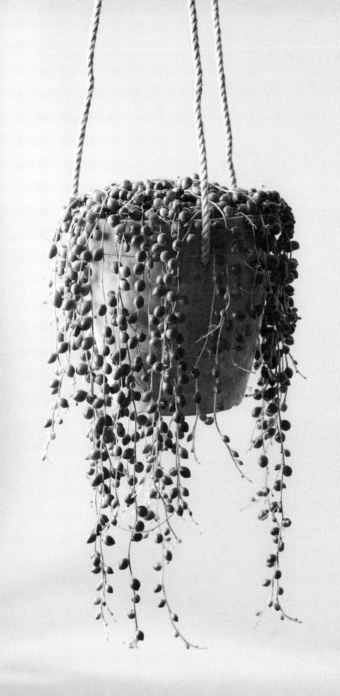

AVOCADO
PERSEA GRATISSIMA

— avocado stone
— 4 toothpicks
— glass jar

+ **CARE** Keep in a warm dry place and top up the water as necessary. After three to four weeks a tap root should emerge, followed by smaller fibrous roots. The stone will split and a shoot should, then soon appear. Allow it to grow to about 10cm and to produce a couple of leaves. Remove the toothpicks and pot the whole plant on using multi-purpose compost, in a pot with plenty of room to come half way up the stone for root growth. Keep in bright, indirect light and warm conditions.

Your own small, home-grown avocado tree is very unlikely to reach the state of maturity when it will bear fruit, but that's not the point. Growing an avocado from its stone is about the simple pleasure of raising an exotic-looking houseplant from scratch.

HOW TO

Hold the stone pointed side up and stick the toothpicks around the middle section at even intervals. These act as a frame to hold the stone so will need to be secure: try to insert them to a depth of at least 5mm. Sit the stone onto the rim of the jar and top up with water, making sure that the rounded base of the stone is in the water.

GINGER
ZINGIBER OFFICINALE

— piece of root ginger
— multi-purpose compost
— pot with drainage holes

+ CARE After a few weeks green shoot tips will emerge from the compost. After six to eight months the stems should be long enough to harvest. Left to grow, ginger makes a very pretty houseplant that will be happiest in bright, indirect light and a warm spot.

Ginger is easy to grow at home and without too much effort you could be harvesting the fresh stems in just a few months. These have a mild ginger taste and make a great flavouring for cordials or used as a garnish for Asian dishes. Wait about a year and you can harvest the roots, which will have multiplied. Start with fresh root ginger from your corner shop or supermarket and choose a plump, smooth-skinned piece, preferably with some visible small yellow tips from which the stems will grow (these are known as eyes). Pot this up and in a few months you will have a handsome houseplant.

HOW TO

Plant the ginger root so that the eyes are just level with the surface of the compost. Water well, cover the pot with a clear plastic bag and place in a warm, sunny spot.

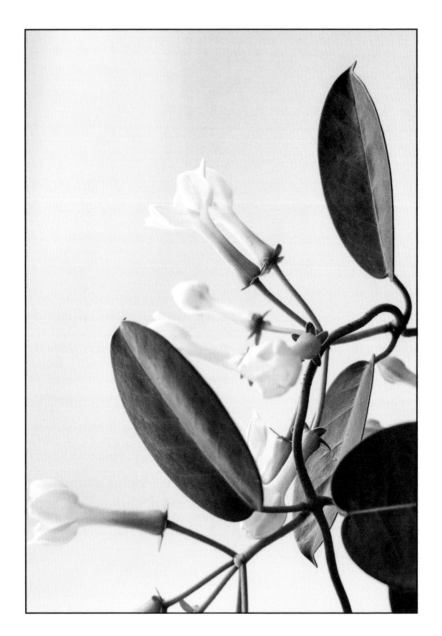

PLANTS THAT BRING JOY AND HAPPINESS

STEPHANOTIS
STEPHANOTIS FLORIBUNDA

○ **LIGHT** Indirect light or filtered sun.

〰 **HUMIDITY** Moderate; stand in a tray of damp pebbles and mist regularly.

◊ **WATERING** Keep the compost damp in the summer and then reduce watering in winter.

✛ **CARE** Apply a high-potash fertilizer once a week when in bud and flowering – usually from spring to autumn.

Scent has been shown to stimulate our emotions. If you have holiday memories of fragrant plants in exotic locations, the perfume of the Stephanotis flower will take you straight back to that happy place. Originating in Madagascar, this semi-tropical vine adapts well to life as a houseplant in cooler climates. Given a trellis or wire support, its long twining stems will clamber up the walls of a sun-room or conservatory.

MARIMO WATER GARDEN

○ **LIGHT** Keep out of direct sun, which will turn the moss ball brown. Marimo will photosynthesise in normal household light.

◊ **WATER** — Change the water every one or two weeks; more regularly in warm weather. Bottled or tap water is fine.

✛ **CARE** In their natural habitat the balls are gently rotated along the floor of the lake by currents and this helps to preserve their roundness. If your Marimo is losing its shape, gently agitate the water so it will settle back on the bottom on a different side. Marimo grow very slowly, gaining just 5mm a year.

What looks like a beautiful moss ball is actually a form of algae, found growing naturally in the pure waters of two lakes – Akan in Japan and Myvatn in Iceland. According to tradition, a gift of Marimo will ensure both the giver and receiver get their heart's desire. The green balls represent enduring love that will weather time and tribulations.

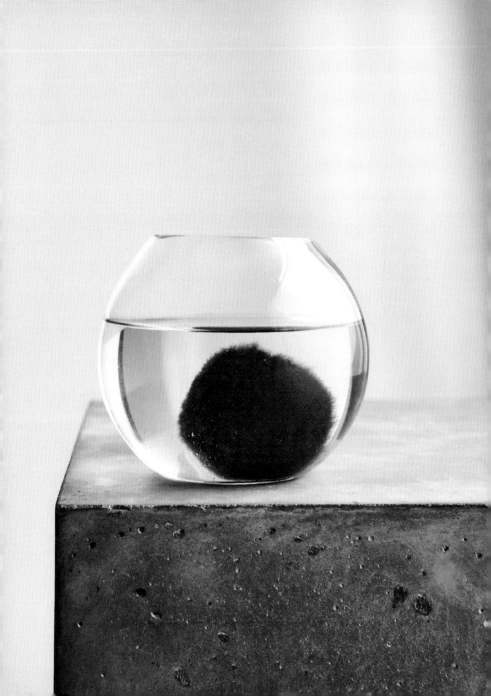

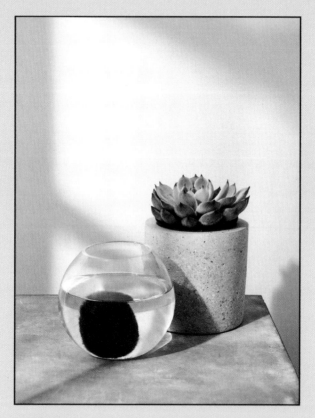

ECHEVERIA AND MARIMO WATER GARDEN

Plants

for the

<u>workspace</u>

Workplaces that feature green plants have been shown to boost productivity and increase staff well-being. So-called 'sick building syndrome' results from poorly ventilated buildings where airborne contaminants, such as moulds and bacteria, thrive if humidity levels are too low or too high. If space is limited, choose small desktop plants like the African Spear (*Sansevieria cylindrica*), some cacti, or let a String of Pearls (*Senecio rowleyanus*) trail from a shelf. If there is plenty of natural light and space go for bold, floor-standing plants that will add character and an exotic ambience to the space.

ECHEVERIA

ECHEVERIA

○ **LIGHT** Sun or filtered light.

〰 **HUMIDITY** Low.

◊ **WATERING** Allow the compost to dry out between watering in the summer. The plants will become dormant in winter so minimal watering is needed.

✚ **CARE** A tiny plant in a mini-pot will dry out very quickly. Grouping a few plants together in one larger pot or terrarium will look great and keeps maintenance to a minimum.

One boring cactus can easily be overlooked but a collection of cacti in fun pots will give your desk space personality. There are hundreds of species, each with a distinctive appeal, and they make perfect office plants. As long as they are placed in a bright sunny spot, cacti and succulents can withstand any amount of neglect; you are much more likely to kill them with kindness, so keep watering to a minimum.

These pretty succulents store water in their juicy, rosette-shaped leaves that may be lilac, grey, pink, smooth or downy, rounded or pointed. Available in a massive range of colours, textures and shapes, they are often sold as mini-plants in tiny pots.

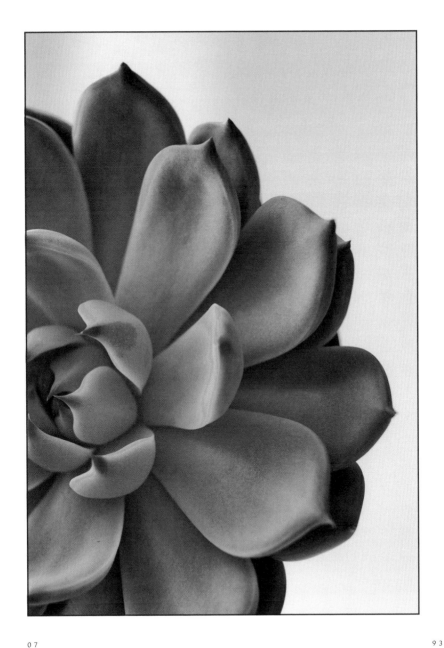

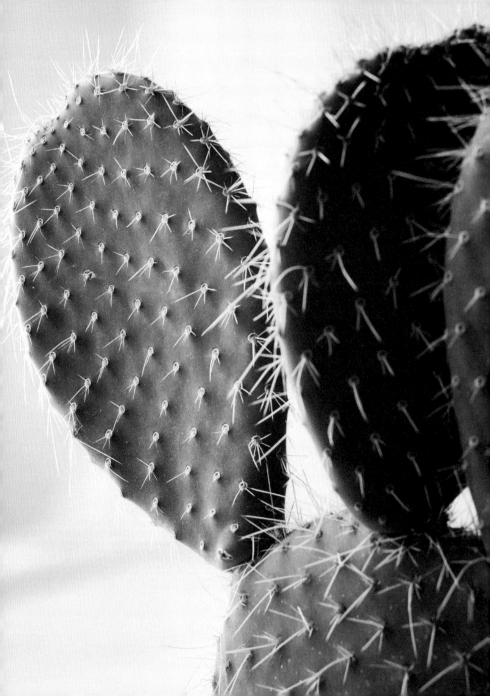

BUNNY EARS
OPUNTIA MICRODASYS

○ **LIGHT** Full or filtered sun.

≋ **HUMIDITY** Low.

◊ **WATERING** Water weekly in summer when light levels are high. In winter, water just once or twice then more regularly in spring.

+ **CARE** Place in a cooler room in winter. Bring back into a warmer spot in spring to encourage flowering.

This cactus may looks like a cartoon bunny but just don't stroke its ears! The flat pads are covered in fine hairs known as glochids that attach themselves to your fingers very easily and feel like mini-splinters. They can irritate your skin and will need to be removed with tweezers. Handle with care and in the summer you will be rewarded with yellow bowl-shaped flowers. See image opposite.

ZEBRA ALOE
HAWORTHIA ATTENUATA

○ **LIGHT** Filtered light.

≋ **HUMIDITY** Low.

◊ **WATERING** In summer allow the compost to dry out between watering and in the winter water very sparingly.

+ **CARE** The leaves will turn brown if placed in direct sunlight.

These very compact and very slow-growing succulents are perfect for those of us who are tight on space. They will get by quite happily provided they are kept warm and out of direct sunlight.

FISHBONE CACTUS
EPIPHYLLUM ANGULIGER

○ **LIGHT** Filtered sun or light shade.

〜 **HUMIDITY** Moderate; loves regular misting.

◊ **WATERING** Water regularly between spring and autumn but ensure the compost dries out between watering. Keep quite dry in winter, watering only occasionally.

+ **CARE** Move the plant to a cooler space in winter to encourage flowering the following autumn. The lovely pale-yellow flowers have a delicious fragrance.

When you've run out of desk space, make full use of any vertical space with pots on shelves or hanging macramé holders. This beautiful forest cactus makes an elegant hanging plant but prefers to be kept out of direct sunlight.

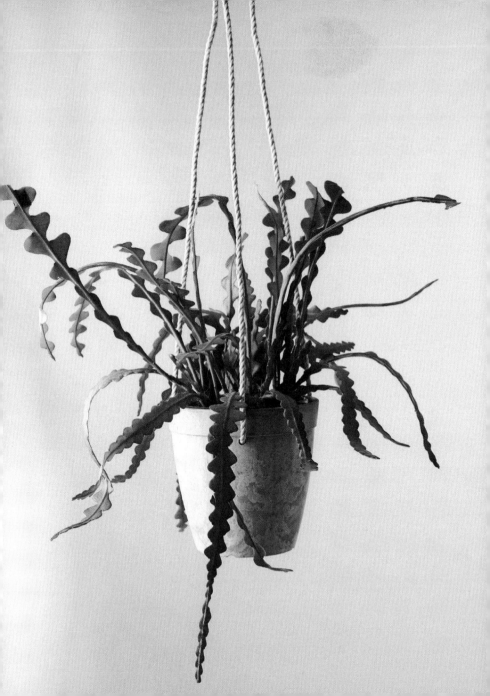

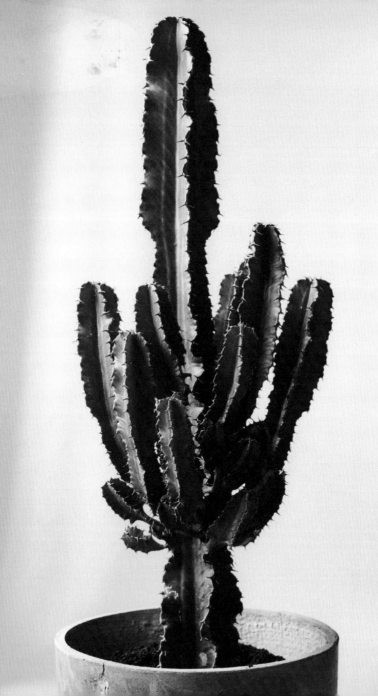

COWBOY CACTUS
EUPHORBIA INGENS

○ LIGHT Bright.

≈ HUMIDITY Low.

◊ WATERING Water moderately when in growth over the summer months. Reduce significantly in the dormant period over winter to just a couple of waterings.

+ CARE The milky sap within the branching stems of this euphorbia is highly toxic if ingested. It may also cause a skin rash on contact.

This statuesque cactus will potentially grow quite large. Start it off on your desk but be prepared to move it to a suitably sunny spot when it starts to take up too much space.

UMBRELLA PLANT
SCHEFFLERA ARBORICOLA

○ **LIGHT** Prefers bright, indirect light but can tolerate lower light levels. Keep out of hot direct sun.

〰 **HUMIDITY** Moderate but can tolerate drier conditions.

◊ **WATERING** Allow the surface of the compost to dry out between watering and make sure that water can drain easily out of the pot. Yellowing leaves indicate overwatering.

✛ **CARE** Re-pot every two years in the spring. In low light conditions the plant may become leggy but can be tip-pruned to encourage bushy growth.

This remarkably easy-going plant is perfect for the workspace because it adapts so well to life in our centrally heated and air-conditioned buildings. Although it can survive a little neglect, it is handsome with glossy palmate leaves and deserves to be well cared for. Follow the guidelines below and you will be rewarded with a healthy, fast-growing plant.

ZZ PLANT

ZAMIOCULCAS ZAMIIFOLIA

○ **LIGHT** Prefers filtered light or light shade but can tolerate most light conditions.

〰 **HUMIDITY** Low.

◊ **WATERING** During the summer months water sparingly and only when the top of the compost has dried out. In winter water once a month.

+ **CARE** To maintain a compact shape, trim back any stems that may have become a little leggy. This is best done in spring.

A work-place hero on many levels, the ZZ is a really tough plant that will tolerate neglect, shady conditions or bright light, and low humidity. It is an excellent air cleaner helping to remove toxins such as xylene and benzene (found in solvents, inks and paint) that may be contributing to nausea and headaches at work. The ZZ Plant is also an effective oxygenator and can improve the quality of the indoor atmosphere.

CAST IRON PLANT
ASPIDISTRA ELATIOR

○ **LIGHT** Light shade or shade.

≋ **HUMIDITY** Low.

◊ **WATERING** Water only when the top of the compost has dried out completely. Reduce watering in winter.

+ **CARE** Feed once in summer to encourage new leaves. Repot every two to three years.

The name says it all. This is one tough cookie of a plant that is ideal for that draughty, shaded spot in the office where nothing else will grow. It's not the most exciting plant to look at, but the leaves have a certain bold, architectural appeal and there are some varieties with variegated splashes, stripes or spots.

FIDDLE-LEAF FIG
FICUS LYRATA

○ **LIGHT** Bright but filtered light.

≋ **HUMIDITY** High; likes regular misting.

◊ **WATERING** Allow the compost to dry out between watering in the summer and keep just moist in winter.

+ **CARE** Easy to look after as long as you don't overwater or allow the pot to sit in water. This will cause root rot.

This tropical rainforest tree, like other figs, makes a good-sized houseplant that will blur the boundaries between outdoors and in. The large leaves are not only great for absorbing pollutants from the air and for humidity control, but they also absorb noise. This is the ideal plant for reducing background office chatter. If space is a little tight, choose the more compact 'Bambino' form. See image opposite.

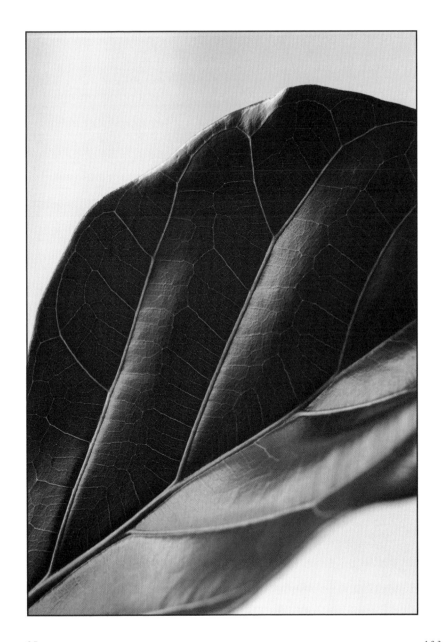

KENTIA PALM
HOWEA FORSTERIANA

○ LIGHT Prefers semi-shade.

〰 HUMIDITY Moderate;
mist every few days.

◊ WATERING Between
spring and autumn water
only when the top of the
compost is dry. Reduce
watering in winter.

+ CARE Feed with a liquid
fertilizer every two weeks
in the summer. The edges
of the leaves may turn
brown if the plant is kept in
a draught or near a radiator.

Large-leaved plants, including palms, naturally
control humidity levels: they release more water
through transpiration when relative humidity
is low and decrease the rate of transpiration
when humidity levels are high. Humidity levels
indoors play an important role in health: too
low and you are more likely to catch a cold or
flu; too high and there is increased likelihood
of moulds and mildew. Dust mites also multiply
faster in high-humidity environments. The
shade-loving Kentia Palm can reach 2.5 metres
and will make the perfect focal point in a dim
corner of the office.

SWORD FERN
NEPHROLEPIS EXALTATA

○ **LIGHT** Prefers bright indirect light but is also tolerant of light shade.

≈ **HUMIDITY** Moderate.

◊ **WATERING** Keep the compost wet throughout the summer months but do not allow to sit in water. Allow the compost to dry out between watering in winter.

+ **CARE** Keep out of direct sunlight and draughts. In cooler months keep away from radiators; this may cause leaf drop.

The Sword Fern is closely related to the Boston Fern and is equally good at removing toxins from indoor air. In tests, this delicate little plant was top of the class when it came to clearing the air of toluene, a solvent found in paint, glue, adhesives and cleaning products. Toluene can cause respiratory problems and is particularly aggravating to asthma sufferers. Unlike the Boston Fern, this plant is more tolerant of the often-dry office atmosphere and being quite compact, it will fit neatly on your desk.

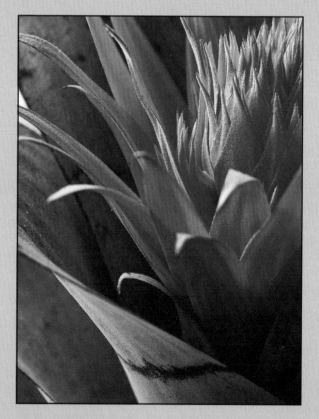

URN PLANT

Plants to help you <u>get well</u> soon

Plants enhance the healing environment. According to studies, hospital patients with plants in their rooms feel more positive, have lower blood pressure and reduced stress levels. The introduction of plants into hospitals has been shown to decrease symptoms of ill health by 25 per cent. Just being in close proximity to plants boosts feelings of calm and aids faster recovery from injury. And when surrounded by plants, some people have a reduced dependency on painkillers.

BIRD'S NEST FERN
ASPLENIUM NIDUS

○ **LIGHT** Filtered sun or light shade.

〰 **HUMIDITY** Moderate to high; will benefit from misting every few days.

◊ **WATERING** Keep the compost moist but not waterlogged.

\+ **CARE** Feed with a balanced liquid fertilizer every two weeks during the summer months.

Headaches, sore eyes and throat, skin complaints and an increase in airborne viral transmissions can often be attributed to a dry atmosphere. Good levels of humidity in winter are especially important owing to the drying effects of heating systems. Low relative humidity is also known to exacerbate the symptoms of patients with respiratory problems.

If you are recovering from an illness at home you can increase the indoor humidity levels by including the Bird's Nest Fern in a group of similar shade-loving ferns. Place them in a decorative bowl filled with damp pebbles and they will act as natural humidifiers.

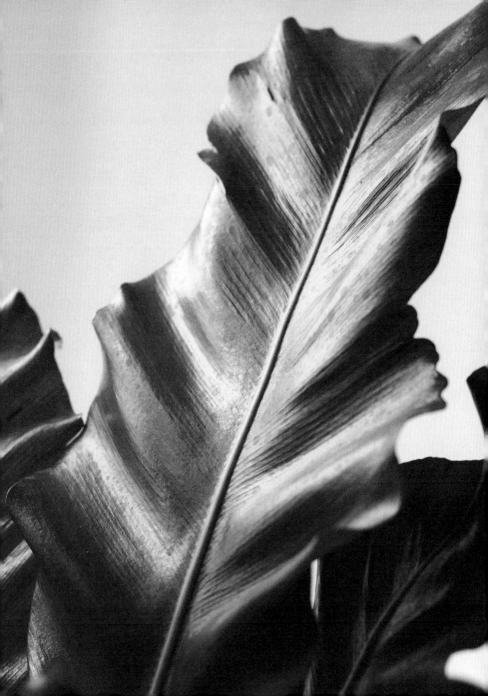

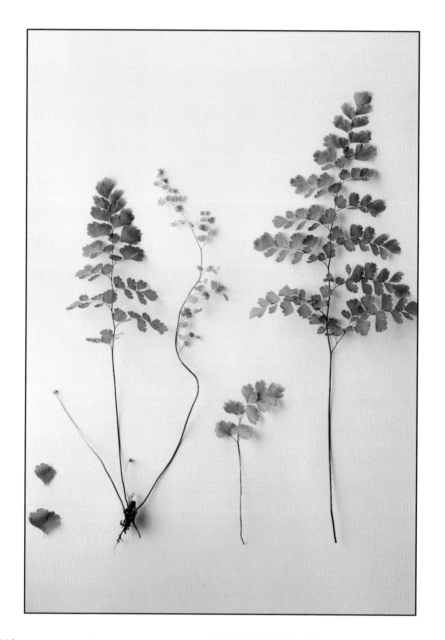

PLANTS TO HELP YOU GET WELL SOON

MAIDENHAIR FERN
ADIANTUM RADDIANUM

○ **LIGHT** Filtered light or light shade.

〰 **HUMIDITY** Moderate to high; sit on a tray of damp pebbles or mist daily.

◊ **WATERING** Do not allow the compost to dry out; keep it moist at all times.

+ **CARE** If the plant does dry out, sit the pot in a sink full of water until the compost is fully soaked. Any tatty or browning stems can be cut back to the base in spring; new growth will soon appear.

One of the prettiest ferns around, the Maidenhair is also one of the most difficult to keep alive unless you can offer it high humidity, regular watering and a spot well out of a draught. It is going to be far happier and more likely to survive if grouped together with other moisture- and shade-loving ferns and displayed in a steamy bathroom.

EMERALD FERN
ASPARAGUS
DENSIFLORUS SPRENGERI

○ **LIGHT** Filtered sun or light shade.

〣 **HUMIDITY** Moderate to high; will benefit from misting every few days.

◊ **WATERING** Keep the compost moist but not waterlogged.

✛ **CARE** Re-pot in the spring if the plant has become root-bound.

This delicate-looking little fern is actually very tough. The gently arching stems resemble plumes and can grow quite long. Display it in a hanging pot or place it on a high shelf.

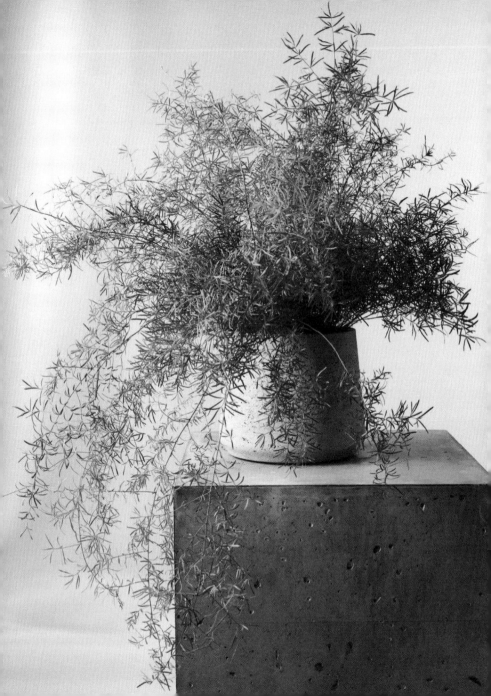

URN PLANT
AECHMEA FASCIATA

○ **LIGHT** Indirect light or light shade.

〰 **HUMIDITY** Moderate.

◊ **WATERING** Keep the central 'urn' made by the leaves (usually known as the plant's 'tank') topped up with water.

✛ **CARE** Empty the tank and rinse your bromeliad at least once a month. Do this more often if you notice build-up on the leaves. Filling the tank with distilled water or rainwater will help prevent the build up of deposits left by tap water.

A beautiful bromeliad from Brazil, the Urn Plant has silver foliage and a neon-pink flower spike. Group it with other forest-dwelling plants with lush green leaves, such as *Monstera* and *Philodendron*, to set off its spectacular foliage. Bromeliads are known to filter out harmful VOCs (volatile organic compounds) from the air, particularly acetone (found in nail polish and household cleaners) which may exacerbate asthma symptoms.

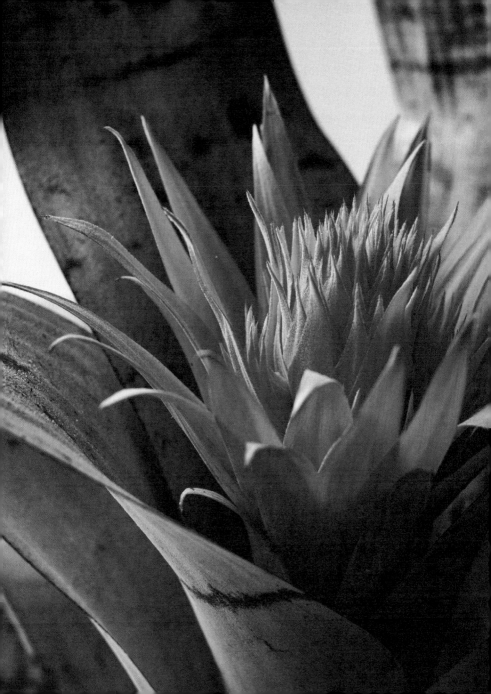

ALOE

ALOE VERA

○ LIGHT Bright light or filtered sun.

〜 HUMIDITY Low.

◊ WATERING From spring to autumn water only once a fortnight; in winter keep the compost almost dry.

+ CARE The leaves may brown and scorch in full sun so move it slightly away from the window in the summer months. You can pot on the young offsets that grow near the parent plant to increase your stock (see Propagation p.172.)

Many of us know about the medicinal uses of this beautiful, fleshy leaved, architectural plant. The clear gel in the leaves is packed full of vitamins, enzymes, amino acids and other compounds that are effective for wound healing and burns. The gel has antibacterial and anti-inflammatory properties. The Aloe's air-purifying abilities are less well known and it is one of the best plants for removing formaldehyde from the air in your home. It will sit happily on a sunny windowsill and is extremely tolerant of neglect. Aloes hold moisture in their thick succulent leaves so go easy on the watering. Every kitchen should have an Aloe as a first-aid remedy for minor burns or sunburn. Simply cut a lower leaf back to the stem and apply the gel to the burn. After application, wrap the leaf in clingfilm and keep in the fridge for up to two weeks.

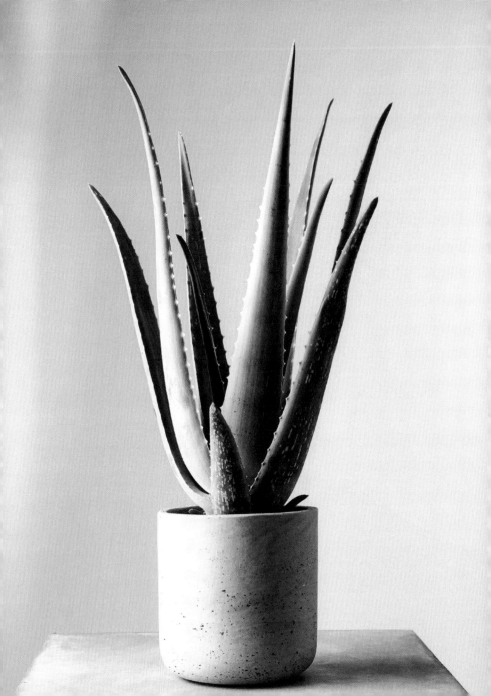

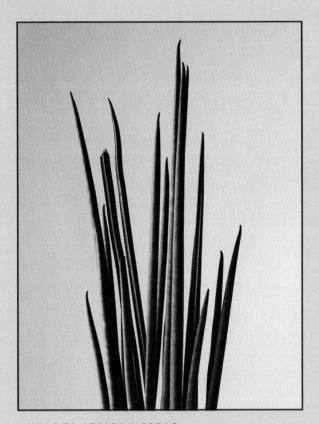

'MIKADO' AFRICAN SPEAR

Plants can help to reduce mental fatigue. The reason most of us can stare at the screen for only so long is that we have a limited capacity for this kind of work, known as directed attention. Contrast this with the undirected attention that is engaged while walking in the park. You might glance up at a group of trees, or closely examine the veining on a leaf. Undirected attention is effortless and allows the directed attention system to rest in preparation for the next bout of screen work. You may not have time to take a walk in the park so recreate its green environment by arranging plants around your workspace.

Plants to boost brain power and focus

CROTON
CODIAEUM VARIEGATUM

○ **LIGHT** Bright,
indirect light.

〟 **HUMIDITY** High; sit
the pot in a tray of damp
pebbles to maintain high
humidity. This method
is preferable to misting
the leaves.

◊ **WATERING** Use tepid
water keep the compost
moist at all times throughout
the spring and summer.
Allow the compost to dry
out between watering in
the winter.

✛ **CARE** Keep the plant out
of draughts and with
constant warmth, but away
from heaters. Don't let the
temperature fall below 15ºC.

Tests have shown that when completing tasks
in an environment where there are living plants,
compared to one devoid of nature, the work
is completed to a higher standard and is more
accurate. But you don't have to go outside to
enjoy dramatic, colourful foliage. The highly
patterned, rainbow-coloured leaves of the
Croton echo the changing hues of autumn.
Crotons have a reputation of being slightly
tricky plants and they certainly don't react
well to change or disruption. The journey
home from the shop may be enough to put
the plant into shock and cause leaf drop. But
persevere; once settled in a warm and humid
spot, the leaves will re-grow.

LIVING STONES
LITHOPS

○ **LIGHT** Bright, sunny conditions; aim for four to five hours of bright light each day.

≋ **HUMIDITY** Low.

◊ **WATERING** Plants are dormant in summer, so water very sparingly from spring to late summer. In the early autumn increase watering to keep the leaves plump.

+ **CARE** In late autumn, a flower should emerge from between the leaves and when this fades, a new set of leaves will emerge from the small fissure. At this point stop watering the plant completely: it will take all the moisture and nutrients it needs from the old leaves as they decay.

Having a few small pots of these curious plants on your desk allows for an easy fix of undirected attention. Take a moment out from your work to examine the detail of these small and truly fascinating succulents, which have evolved to blend in with the surrounding rocks. This clever characteristic prevents them from being eaten by hungry desert herbivores.

MINT
MENTHA

○ **LIGHT** Bright, sunny spot.

≈ **HUMIDITY** Low.

◊ **WATERING** Soak the compost thoroughly but allow it to dry out completely before watering again.

+ **CARE** Move outdoors in summer: Pinch off any flowers; these will divert the plant's energy away from the leaves.

There are many varieties of this familiar herb and in all of them the scent is naturally stimulating. It can help to boost energy levels as well as lift our mood. Release the natural oils by rubbing the leaves between your fingers and inhale the scent deeply. If you're feeling a bit sluggish, make a refreshing tea with a few leaves plucked from the plant. This is best done in the morning when the oil concentration is at its strongest.

ROSEMARY
ROSMARINUS OFFICINALIS

○ **LIGHT** Strong sunlight.

≈ **HUMIDITY** Low.

◊ **WATERING** Give the plant a good soak and then allow to dry out completely before watering again.

+ **CARE** Prefers a gritty, free-draining compost; never allow the pot to sit in water. Pinch out the tips of the stems to encourage a bushy habit.

Compounds found in this familiar culinary herb have been shown to improve brain function: the smell alone can enhance our ability to remember complex events and tasks. Although usually grown outside, rosemary will thrive in a pot on the doorstep or on a sunny south facing window sill. To release the powerful scent, rub the leaves between your fingers and inhale deeply. Small molecules of the plant's essential oil will pass into the bloodstream and from there to the brain.

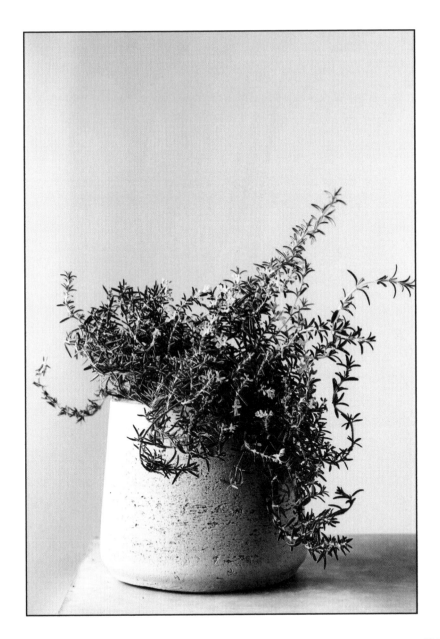

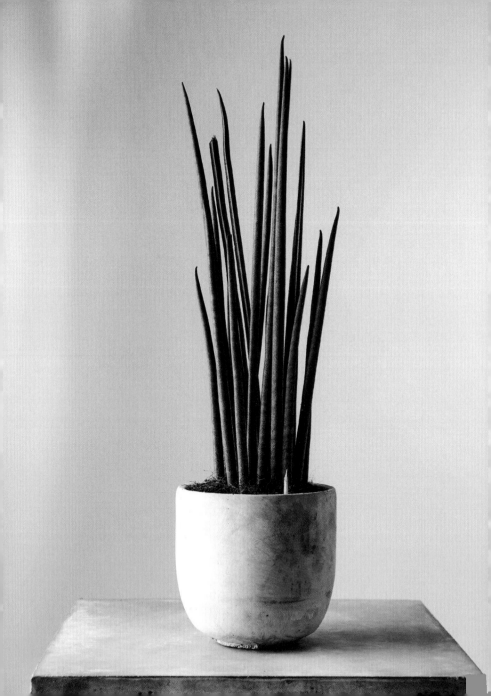

'MIKADO' AFRICAN SPEAR
SANSEVIERIA BACULARIS

○ LIGHT Prefers filtered
sun or light shade but
can tolerate most
light conditions.

〰 HUMIDITY Low.

◊ WATERING Sparingly;
allow the compost to dry
out completely between
watering in summer months.
Reduce frequency to about
once a month in winter.

✛ CARE This plant prefers
to have its roots constricted
so when re-potting choose
a pot that is no more than
5cm larger in diameter
than the root ball. Use
a free-draining cactus
compost or add bark chips
to multi-purpose compost.

Studying in the presence of plants can deepen
concentration and may also improve memory. If
you have a lot of information to digest, it's worth
making space for plants on your desk, such as
this small and compact *Sansevieria*. Tough and
resilient, this is a plant that can withstand a
certain amount of drought as well as shady
or bright conditions.

BAMBOO PALM
RHAPIS EXCELSA

○ **LIGHT** Light shade or shade.

≀≀ **HUMIDITY** Low to moderate; mist the leaves throughout the summer.

◊ **WATERING** Water well between spring and autumn but ensure the plant is not waterlogged and allow the top of the compost to dry out between watering. Reduce watering in winter.

✛ **CARE** Will tolerate deep shade in summer but may need to be moved nearer to a window in winter when light levels drop.

Large plants such as the dense Bamboo Palm will help to create a lush, green environment that will aid concentration. One of the easiest palms to grow, it is tolerant of low light and dry air, and although slow growing it can potentially reach 2 metres. As an added benefit, this NASA-recommended plant effectively cleans the air of most commonly found indoor toxins.

PANDA PLANT
KALANCHOE TOMENTOSA

○ LIGHT Filtered sun or indirect bright light.

〰 HUMIDITY Low.

◊ WATERING Water only when the compost has dried out completely and at the base of the pot to avoid damaging the leaves by water splash. Ideally, sit the plant in a tray of water until the top of the compost is moist.

+ CARE The Panda Plant can grow up to 1 metre and form quite a large plant with a tree-like silhouette. The plant is easily propagated with leaf cuttings (see Propagation p.174)

Richly deserving of space on your desk, this velvet-leaved, tactile little plant demands to be stroked. The simple act of touching the soft, smooth surface of the leaf can also reduce feelings of stress. When you are under pressure and in need of distraction, keep this plant nearby and give yourself a quick, calming fix. (See image p.175.)

RUBBER PLANT
FICUS ELASTICA

○ **LIGHT** Filtered, indirect light; direct sun will scorch the leaves.

〜 **HUMIDITY** Mist frequently with cool water in warmer months.

◊ **WATERING** Water only when the top of the compost has dried out in the summer. Keep the plant just moist in winter.

╋ **CARE** To maintain a good shape, prune your plant in the spring. Re-pot every two to three years to prevent the plant from becoming pot bound. Keep out of draughts and avoid large fluctuations in temperature – both can cause the leaves to drop.

This beautiful indoor tree is happiest when grouped with other large plants, such as palms or a *Monstera*, as part of a plant 'gang' to help maintain atmospheric humidity within the room. If you treat this fast-growing fig with the care and attention it deserves, it will soon shoot up and make a dramatic statement. Gazing at its exotic greenery will be restorative and allow you to re-focus on the task in hand.

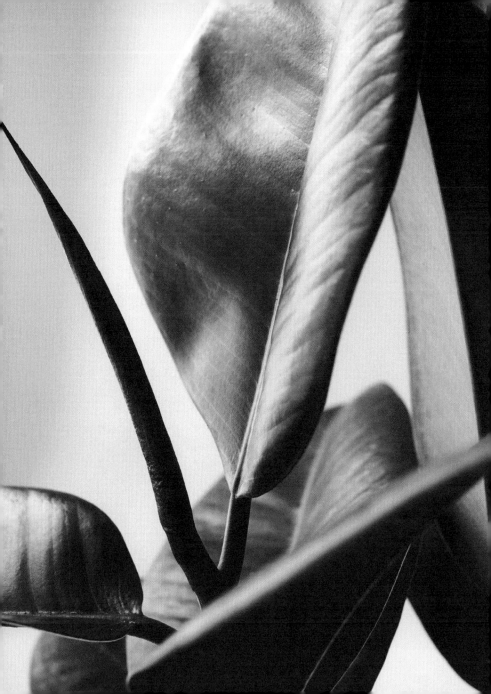

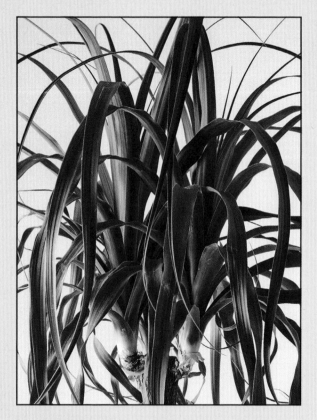

PONYTAIL PALM

Plants to help you communicate and relate

Surround your self with plants to improve interpersonal relationships. It is said that those who spend time around plants enjoy better relationships with people. Feelings of compassion can be increased as a result of being in the company of plants, and people who spend time caring for nature are more likely to care for others. Increasing your collection (see Propagation, p.167) is easy to do and sharing your plants is a great way of making connections with friends and colleagues.

PASS IT ON PLANT
PILEA PEPEROMIOIDES

○ **LIGHT** Bright, indirect light.

⁀ **HUMIDITY** Moderate to high.

◊ **WATERING** Keep moist during spring and summer but don't let the plant sit in water. In winter, allow the surface of the compost to become dry before watering.

✚ **CARE** Spring is the best time to propagate your *Pilea* as the warmth and light will encourage new root and leaf growth; the whole process will take longer in the winter. Rotate your plant every so often so all sides receive equal amounts of light. Mature specimens can become a little straggly and top heavy – a good reason to raise new, more compact plants.

Native to China, this compact plant is easy to care for and will feel at home in your bedroom, bathroom or office. As the common name suggests, this plant readily produces offspring so is made for sharing. When small plantlets sprout up through the compost, carefully separate them from the parent plant and pot them on.

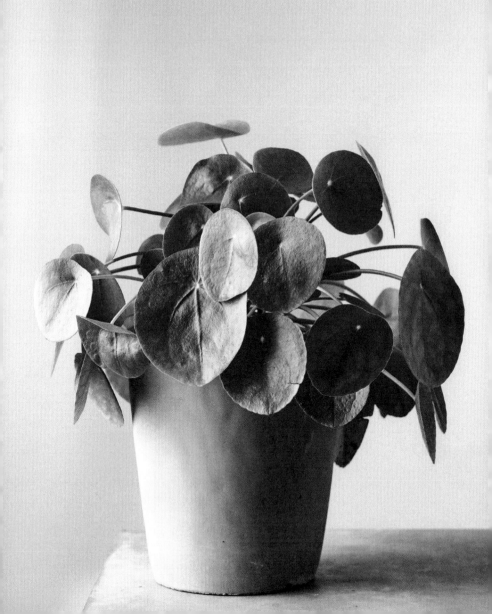

BRAZILIAN BUTTERFLY
OXALIS TRIANGULARIS

○ LIGHT Bright, indirect light.

〰 HUMIDITY Moderate.

◊ WATERING Allow the surface of the compost to dry out between watering. Water only occasionally in winter.

+ CARE When grown from bulb divisions, this plant will become dormant in the winter months and the foliage will die back naturally. Remove the pot to a cool room and stop watering. In the warmer spring months new shoots will start to appear. At this point you can return the plant to its usual spot and resume watering.

The delicate, shamrock-like leaves of this pretty plant move in response to light – folding up at night and unfurling again in the sunlight. It is related to wood sorrel and both the leaves and the small pink flowers are edible; they have a slight citrus flavour. If you pick the flowers they'll keep coming all summer. The plant grows from a 'clump' of small bulbs that is easy to divide.

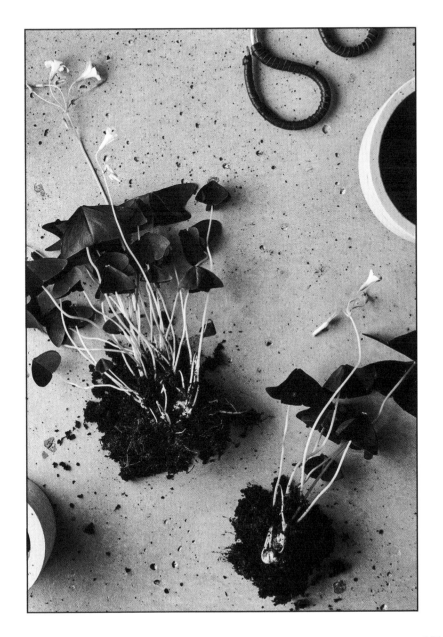

PONYTAIL PALM

BEAUCARNEA RECURVATA

○ **LIGHT** Bright,
sunny position.

〰 **HUMIDITY** Low.

◊ **WATERING** In summer
water about once a week,
allowing the surface of
the compost to dry out
completely between
watering. In winter the
compost should be kept
almost dry.

+ **CARE** The water-holding
stem should provide
sufficient moisture in
both mature and young
specimens to allow the plant
to last through the winter
dormant period. Keep the
plant out of cold draughts.

The bulbous, water-storing trunk of this palm
has the texture and shape of an elephant's foot
– its other common name. Topped by a cascade
of delicate fronds, this unusual plant can grow
to 1 metre and makes a striking specimen. As
the plant matures it reproduces via small shoots
from the base of the trunk: these are the offsets
or pups. They are easily removed and with a little
care can be potted on to grow roots of their own.

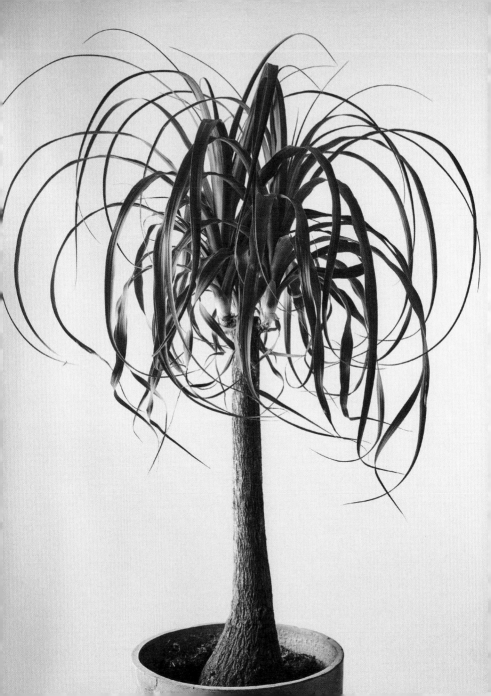

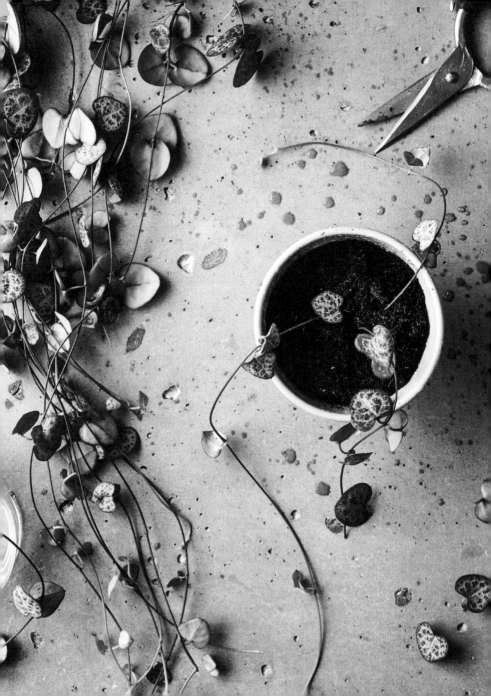

STRING OF HEARTS
CEROPEGIA WOODII

○ **LIGHT** Filtered light, out of direct sun.

〉〉〉 **HUMIDITY** Low.

◊ **WATERING** As a rule of thumb, water only when the top of the compost feels dry and reduce watering in the winter.

✛ **CARE** The plant will not tolerate being over-watered.

Growing at a speedy rate, this lovely trailing plant has superior water-storing tubers that develop along the stem and roots during periods of drought. The tubers can be cut from the plant and potted on, but taking stem cuttings is more convenient: like hair, this fast-growing plant will need a regular trim.

TREE AEONIUM
AEONIUM ARBOREUM

○ **LIGHT** Bright, sunny position.

))) **HUMIDITY** Low.

◊ **WATERING** Give the compost a good soak when it has fully dried out but never let the plant sit in water. In winter, water very sparingly.

+ **CARE** Keep in a cool, frost-free spot over the winter months, away from radiators.

Like other succulents such as the houseleek *(Sempervivum)*, *Aeoniums* form clusters of fleshy rosettes. They start as compact plants but as they mature the stems can get long and leggy, making the plants a little top heavy. To neaten the plants and to grow young plants to share with friends, simply take stem cuttings. (See image p.171.)

INCH PLANT

TRADESCANTIA ZEBRINA

○ **LIGHT** Bright but out of direct sunlight.

〰 **HUMIDITY** Moderate to high.

◊ **WATERING** Keep the compost moist (but not waterlogged). In winter, water only when the compost is dry.

+ **CARE** Inch Plants can become quite leggy and brittle as they mature but if you regularly pinch out the growing tips, this will promote bushier growth. The pinched-out tips can easily be rooted in water.

The many varieties of *Tradescantia*, including this silver- and purple-striped form, are famously easy to root. Why not fill your shelves with them and create the effect of a living wall? (See image on p. 173.)

POLKADOT BEGONIA
BEGONIA MACULATA

○ **LIGHT** Filtered sun or light shade.

〜 **HUMIDITY** Moderate.

◌ **WATERING** Water weekly in the summer but allow the compost to dry out between watering. The fleshy stems of Begonia will rot easily if waterlogged. Keep on the dry side in winter but if the leaves start to curl it is an indication that the plant is too dry.

✛ **CARE** To maintain humidity in the warmer months, sit the pot on a tray of damp pebbles. Do not mist the leaves as this can encourage mould growth caused by the fungal disease, botrytis. Keep away from radiators and draughts in winter.

The dramatic silver-spotted leaves and cascading trusses of cream flowers make this a highly covetable begonia and it is easily propagated from stem cuttings rooted in water.

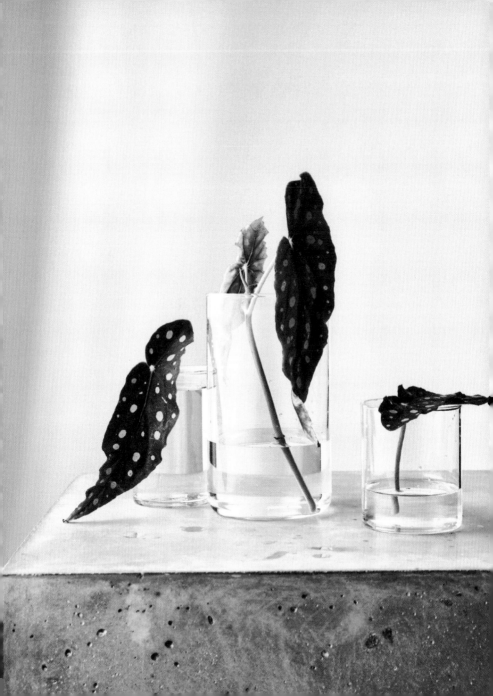

DONKEY'S TAIL
SEDUM MORGANIANUM

○ **LIGHT** Bright sunlight but kepp out of scorching midday sun in summer.

≋ **HUMIDITY** Low.

◊ **WATERING** Moderately throughout the summer, allowing the top of the compost to dry out completely between watering. Water sparingly through the winter.

+ **CARE** When watering, direct the flow to the compost and try not to wet the juicy leaves, which store a lot of water. Overwatering may cause the plant to rot, particularly in the winter.

Handle these pretty succulent plants with care because the leaves are quite brittle and break off easily. A mature plant of six years or more may have stems up to 30cm long, each heavily laden with the plump juicy leaves. Sometimes an overloaded stem can break off, but the good news is that it will take root easily. One mature stem can be divided into sections and will make up to six new plants that can be shared with friends.

MOSAIC PLANT
FITTONIA VERSCHAFFELTII

○ **LIGHT** Indirect light /
moderate shade

≀≀ **HUMIDITY** High.

◊ **WATERING** Keep the
compost moist throughout
the year.

✛ **CARE** If not planted in a
terrarium, you can maintain
your Mosaic Plant's humidity
level by placing the pot in
a tray of damp pebbles.
Although the compost
should be kept moist, do
not allow it to become
waterlogged because the
delicate roots will rot. On
the other hand, the leaves
can wilt dramatically if
the compost has been left
very dry for a few days, but
after a good soak the plant
should revive.

This small, humidity-loving plant is perfect
for a bottle garden or terrarium. And once it
has reached 10–15cm in height, you can gently
tease the stems apart to make three or four
divisions, keeping as much root as possible on
each. Combine the new sections with mini-ferns
or mosses and plant them in glass jars to make
living gifts for friends (see Terrarium p.72).

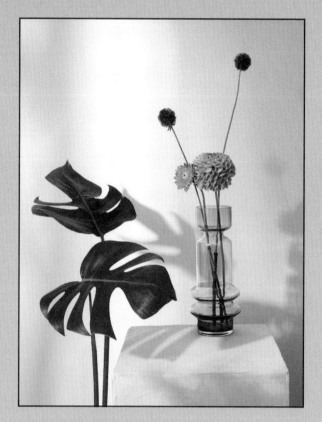

SWISS CHEESE PLANT

CHAPTER 11

How to <u>choose</u> your plants

CHOOSING YOUR PLANTS AND BRINGING THEM HOME

Take the first step to acquiring green fingers by choosing the right plant for your home environment and providing the conditions it needs to grow and thrive. This can be a little intimidating when you start out, but if you find a plant shop or nursery where the staff are trained and can give specialist advice, you will have more chance of success.

First, consider your home environment. How much light and warmth is there? How much space do you have and where do you want to place your plant? Start with plants that are easy to look after, then when you're more confident you can move on to plants that require a little more specialist care. If you have pets or children, consider buying hanging plants that are out of reach of wagging tails and crawling babies.

When you have decided which plant you want to take home with you, have a closer look to try and determine if the plant is healthy. Plants that have been badly cared for are more susceptible to damage from pests and disease and will show the signs of neglect on their leaves and in the compost. The leaves are a particularly good indicator of health: brown patches or yellowing on the leaf indicate that the plant may have a disease or virus. Check the underside of the leaf, too, for pests or damage – small green or white flies, grey mould or powdery mildew are signs of infestation and these plants should be avoided.

Also check for roots growing out of the drainage hole, which is an indication that the plant is pot bound and needs transferring to a larger pot. Although you might be tempted to buy it,

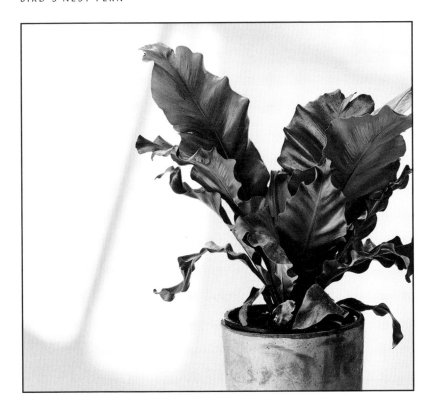

the chances are that the plant will have been weakened due to lack of adequate nutrition and will therefore be more susceptible to disease.

Once your chosen plant has been given the all-clear, take care to wrap it up well for the journey home (tropical houseplants in particular can be damaged by extremes in weather). Protect tropical plants from exposure to the cold in winter and from direct sun in the heat of summer.

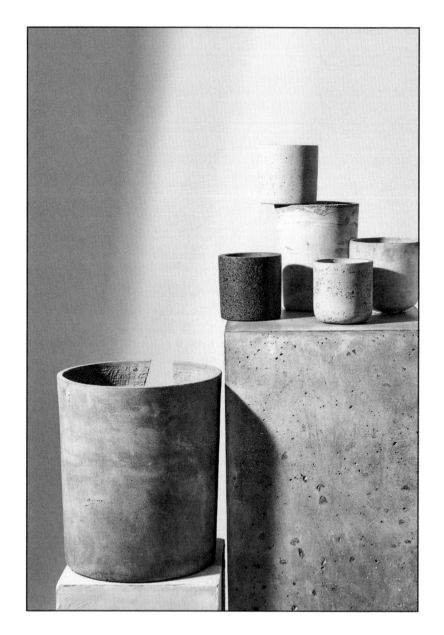

HOW TO CHOOSE YOUR PLANTS

CHOOSING THE CORRECT POT FOR YOUR PLANT

Most houseplants are grown in black plastic pots with drainage holes. While not aesthetically pleasing, this type of pot is the most practical because the plastic retains moisture and the drainage holes prevent the compost from becoming waterlogged. If you want to replace the plastic with a more decorative pot to enhance the foliage and give your plant personality, choose one of a similar size that has drainage holes. But if the new pot lacks drainage holes, you can still use it as an attractive pot cover. Always take the plant in its plastic pot out for watering as required, and allow any excess to drain away before putting it back in the cover.

Once home, your plant needs a settling-in period, a little time to get accustomed to its new surroundings. It is quite normal to see some leaf drop in the first few weeks, but don't be tempted to give additional water or food at this stage – this will just put the plant under more strain. Be patient. Within a few weeks, when the plant has settled down, you should notice signs of new growth.

There's a whole community of plant lovers out there who want to share advice on keeping plants healthy, as well as pass on tips about propagation and ideas for displays. See the directory at the end of this book for a list of useful resources.

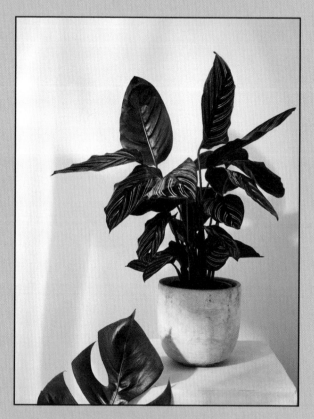

PIN-STRIPE CALATHEA AND SWISS CHEESE

CHAPTER 12

Keeping your plants healthy

Your plants will work harder for you if you keep them in tip-top condition. A healthy plant will be far more effective at removing toxins from the air, for example, than a plant that is struggling to stay alive. And plants that are well cared for are attractive, colourful and satisfying to look at.

It is a good idea to buy your plants from a specialist shop where trained staff will advise you on the best way to care for them. That advice is likely to come not only from experience but also from an understanding of the plant's requirements based on knowledge of its native habitat. Most of our leafy houseplants are native to equatorial rainforest in South America, Asia or Africa, where the climate is typically hot and wet. Under the canopy of the rainforest the plants flourish out of direct sunlight and some of the smaller ground-dwelling plants thrive in quite shaded conditions. These plants generally prefer to be kept in filtered light and a warm, humid atmosphere. Cacti and succulent plants with spines or with water-holding stems and leaves tend to come from arid desert regions where they have adapted to survive hot and dry conditions. This group of plants will need a bright, sunny position and moderate watering to survive.

In their native habitat all these plants have the sun, rain and the earth for light, warmth, water and nutrients – the basic requirements of life. As soon as we put a plant in a pot and bring it into our home it depends on us to provide those basic needs. So when buying plants, always choose specialist plant shops and get the best advice you can. Be kind to your plants and they will love you back.

LIGHT

Basic plant care should start with knowing the ideal light conditions for your plant, then finding the perfect spot in your home to suit its requirements. Skylights that allow light to fall down evenly on to your plants are ideal. South-facing window sills are the brightest and hottest spots, while north-facing ones are the coolest and least bright. Light levels fluctuate between the seasons and light may also be blocked by tall buildings or trees. Take time to identify the light levels in your living space and use this guide to help you find the perfect plant for the perfect place.

SUITABLE PLANTS

Fiddle-Leaf Fig
Fishbone Cactus
Heart Leaf Plant
Pass It On Plant
Prayer Plant
String of Hearts
Swiss Cheese Plant
some cacti and succulents.

PLANTS FOR BRIGHT, INDIRECT LIGHT

These plants prefer to be placed near to a window but out of direct sunlight. Filtered light suits them best, so either position them behind a sheer curtain or at a distance of about 1 metre from a south-facing window. These light conditions are ideal for the majority of large-leaved tropical plants.

SUITABLE PLANTS

Cacti, and succulents
Geranium
Ponytail Palm
Rosemary
Snake Plant

PLANTS FOR DIRECT LIGHT

These plants tend to be desert or Mediterranean dwellers that like to grow in full sun. They will be happiest on a sunny window sill that, in summer, receives over twelve hours of sunlight each day. Some windows have radiators placed beneath them, which can really dry out your plants in the winter months. Those plants that are in their dormant phase, such as cacti and succulents, will need to be moved to a cooler

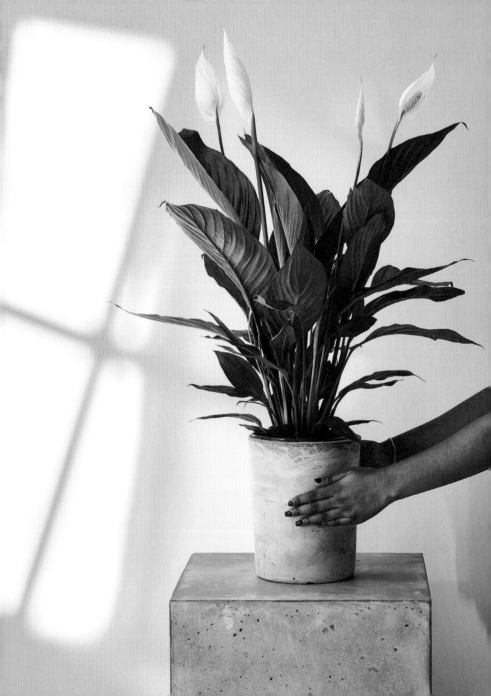

position. Plants that cannot tolerate such bright conditions in summer will enjoy the lower winter light levels and can be put on a window sill until spring.

Bromeliads
Calathea
Chinese Evergreen
Ferns
Ivy
Jade Plant
Parlour Palm
Peace Lily (opposite)
Snake Plant
Spider Plant

PLANTS FOR LIGHT SHADE AND SHADE

These are plants that naturally grow in filtered light or lightly shaded places, such as under the rainforest canopy at the foot of larger trees. They prefer to be out of direct sun, which would scorch their leaves, and generally enjoy damp, humid conditions. Choose a spot in the corner of the room where the hours of sunlight are limited or there is only artificial light. Plants that like shady, damp conditions will often thrive in the humidity of a bathroom or kitchen.

WATERING AND HUMIDITY

Frequency of watering depends on the type of plant and the season. When the weather is warm and light levels are high, plants transpire more quickly and will therefore require more frequent watering. In general, leafy houseplants like a good soak so that the compost is fully wet. The top layer of compost should then be allowed to dry out before watering again. This method is preferable to small top-ups of water every few days, which may cause the plant to become waterlogged. The easiest way to check if the plant is dry is to insert your finger into the top 5cm of compost; if it feels damp, wait until it feels dry before watering again. When you put your hand under hanging plants and they feel light in the pot, this usually means they need watering. Succulent plants and cacti hold water in their leaves and stems and will rot if overwatered, so make sure that the compost dries out completely before watering again. In winter, plant growth slows and many houseplants go into semi-dormancy. This is the time to cut back on watering, particularly with cacti and succulents. Check that your pots have good-sized drainage holes so that excess water can drain away from the roots and never allow your plants to sit in water. This is a common cause of root rot, which will kill them.

Many houseplants are from the tropics and have adapted to thrive in high levels of humidity. To increase humidity levels, mist your plants regularly and group them together. As they transpire, they create a humid microclimate. Ferns and Calathea love to be kept in the humid conditions of a bathroom or kitchen. Cacti and succulents are from arid regions and need warm and dry conditions. (Bird's Nest and *Kokedama* Ferns opposite)

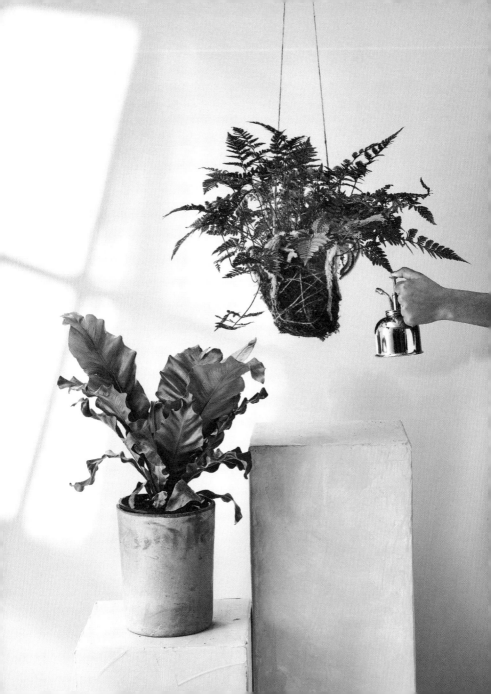

FEEDING

Feeding is only really necessary over the summer months when your plant is in full growth. Plants take up fertilizer through their roots in solution, so dry compost will limit their capacity to absorb nutrients. Most houseplants need a balanced liquid fertilizer containing nitrogen, phosphorus and potassium – this is usually bought as a liquid, or a powder, that you then dilute in water. At, or just before, flowering time, houseplants need a high-potassium feed. Large, woody, tree-like houseplants, on the other hand, benefit from a slow-release granular fertilizer that is applied to the surface of the compost, or inserted in the form of a spike, once a year. Don't be tempted to overfeed your plants as this will have a detrimental effect, producing weak growth and brown tips on the leaves.

RE-POTTING

The classic sign that your plant needs re-potting is when roots are growing out of the drainage hole. Gently tip the plant out of its pot and you will probably notice that the roots are tightly compacted and circling around the inside of the pot. If your plant wilts quickly after watering or if the leaves are pale or yellowing, these are also indications that the plant isn't getting enough nutrients from the soil and needs a bigger pot. As a rough guide, most mature plants will need re-potting once every two to three years; young plants more frequently. The best time of year is late winter or early spring, just when the plant is starting into growth.

Choose a pot no bigger than one size up (usually no more than an extra 5cm in diameter) and with good-sized drainage holes to allow excess water to drain out. Water your plant well about 30 minutes before repotting and then remove the plant from its container. Fill the new pot with a layer of compost – multi-purpose is fine for the majority of plants but you will need specialist compost for cacti, succulents and orchids. Gently tease out the compacted roots to encourage new growth then set the plant into its new pot, with the surface approximately 1cm below the rim. Fill in the gaps with more compost and press it down gently to remove air pockets, making sure the compost isn't compacted, which will prevent oxygen getting to the roots. Water the plant well, letting any excess water drain away before placing it in your chosen spot.

If, however, you have a large plant and you want to restrict its growth, you can do this by pruning back both the stems and the roots. Pruning should be done no more than once a year and it is best carried out in spring, using sharp, clean secateurs. Always prune stems just above a leaf node (the bump on the stem where new growth develops). If your plant has become too tall and you want a more compact plant, you can simply pinch out the growing tip of the stem. This encourages side-shoots and bushier growth lower down the stem.

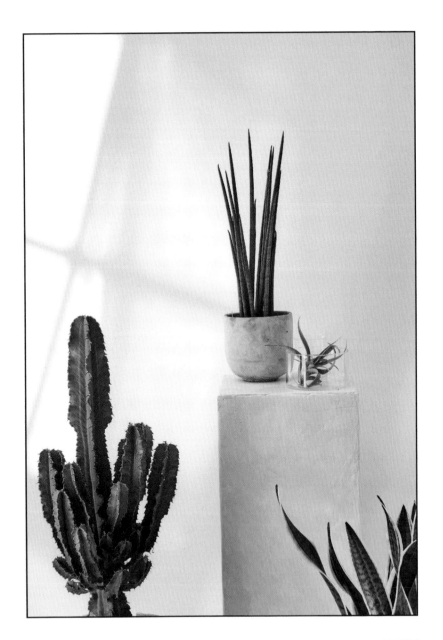

KEEPING YOUR PLANTS HEALTHY

KEEPING
YOUR PLANTS
HEALTHY
WHILE
YOU'RE AWAY

Follow these simple rules and you will return home to happy, hydrated plants:

– Remove plants from window sills: they will become hot and dehydrated from the summer sun. Plants left there in winter will suffer from cold, so move them further away.

– Group your plants together to make a humid microclimate and place humidity-loving plants, such as ferns, in a tray filled with damp pebbles. As the water evaporates it will create a humid atmosphere around the plant.

– If you have a bath, soak a couple of old towels in water and lay them out in it like mats to increase humidity. Group your plants together and place them on the soaking towels so they can take up moisture when they need it.

– If you don't have a bath, fill the kitchen sink with water and place a towel on the draining board with one end sitting in the water. Arrange your plants on the towel, which will soak up moisture and hydrate the plants.

– Make a drip bottle to water larger plants. Cut the bottom off a plastic drinks bottle and make a small hole in the cap with a skewer. Upend the bottle and gently push the cap and neck into the compost. Fill the bottle with water to create a reservoir that will allow the water to drip slowly through to the roots as needed.

('Mikado' African Spear, Cowboy Cactus, Air Plant and Snake Plant opposite.)

PLANTS
AND PETS

It isn't easy convincing your pets to live in harmony with your plants. Puppies, for example, can be trained and if given alternative stimulation, such as pet toys, will soon learn to leave the plants alone. Cats present more of a challenge and indoor cats, in particular, will chew on leaves and bat trailing stems with their paws or knock hanging plants from shelves when they get bored. Outdoor cats eat grass to induce vomiting and clear their stomachs of fur balls and small pieces of bone and feather. If your indoor cat has a taste for greens and is nibbling your plants, sow trays of widely available 'cat grass'. The seeds sprout quickly and within a few weeks your cat will have its own indoor lawn to graze on.

Some of the houseplants profiled in this book are toxic if ingested by animals. The severity of the reaction will depend on the amount of plant eaten and the size of your pet, but the symptoms are usually vomiting and stomach upset.

SUITABLE PLANTS

Bamboo Palm
Boston Fern
Christmas Cactus
Echeveria
Moth Orchid
Parlour Palm
Ponytail Palm
Spider Plant
Urn Plant

SOME PET-FRIENDLY PLANTS

For those of us who have young dogs or cats that like to chew on foliage, the list below identifies the safest houseplants to have in your home.

UNSUITABLE PLANTS

Heart Leaf
Jade Plant
Snake Plant
Swiss Cheese Plant
Umbrella Plant
ZZ Plant

SOME PLANTS FEATURED IN THIS BOOK THAT ARE TOXIC TO PETS

Ingestion of the following plants can cause major irritation in the mouth, vomiting and stomach upset.

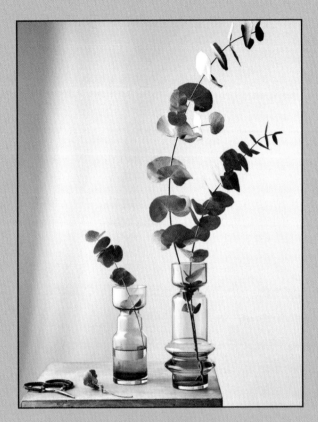

EUCALYPTUS

CHAPTER 13

Plants

to

<u>share</u>

Multiplying your stock is not only free and easy to do but it is also really satisfying to see the young plants that you have propagated grow and thrive in your care. You can then share your love of houseplants by making presents of the young plants to friends and family.

There are five basic techniques for propagating houseplants: offsets, division, stem in compost, stem in water and leaf cuttings. The different methods, which are suited to different plants depending on their structure and natural habit, are described overleaf.

1 OFFSETS

+ **CARE** When watering, direct the flow to the compost and try not to wet the juicy leaves, which store a lot of water. Overwatering may cause the plant to rot, particularly in the winter.

SUITABLE PLANTS

Bromeliads
Pass It On Plant
Ponytail Palm
Spider Plant
Succulents such as Aloe Vera

This is the easiest method of propagation for any plants that produce offsets. These small plants (sometimes known as 'pups') grow around the base of the parent plant and can simply be detached and grown on in small pots.

HOW TO

Choose a strong-growing offset about 5–10cm in length. Either use a sharp knife to sever the offset or remove the parent plant from its pot and gently disentangle the roots of the young plant. Whichever method you use, try to retain as much root as possible. Fill a small pot with suitable compost, make a hole with a pencil or dibber, put the plant in, firm gently and dampen the compost lightly. Keep the young plant out of direct sunlight. After a few weeks the roots will grow, anchoring the plant into the pot.

2 DIVISION

+ CARE Water the compost
and set the plants in a
bright, warm spot out of
direct sun. Make sure not to
overwater or feed at this
stage: the young plants will
need a rest period after the
shock of being separated.
Given time and a little water,
the plants will start to grow
and thrive.

SUITABLE PLANTS

African Spear Plant
Brazilian Butterfly Plant
Cast Iron Plant
Mosaic Plant
Peace Lily
Pin-Stripe Calathea
Sword Fern and most
other ferns
Urn Plant

Suitable for most multi-stemmed plants,
division will give a new lease of life to mature
plants that have become overcrowded in the
pot. Houseplants are best divided in spring,
giving them a chance to recover over the
summer growing period.

HOW TO

Water the plant you want to divide and leave for
at least 30minutes to drain. Remove the plant
from its pot and gently tease apart the clump
into two or even three sections, ensuring plenty
of root remains attached to each. Very mature
plants can be difficult to divide and you may
need a sharp knife to cut through and separate
congested roots. Fill new pots with suitable
compost and plant the divisions into the pots
at the same level as they were previously. Take
care not to damage the roots.

3 STEM CUTTINGS IN COMPOST

CARE Keep new plants in a bright spot but out of full sun and check for signs of new growth every week or two. Once new leaves emerge, remove the plastic covering.

SUITABLE PLANTS

Figs
String of Hearts
Swiss Cheese Plant
Tree Aeonium (opposite)

This easy way of making new plants is often the most successful and is suitable for most soft-stemmed plants. It is best to take cuttings in the spring or summer – the plant's natural growing season. Dusting the end of the cutting with hormone rooting powder will help speed up the process but is not essential for success.

HOW TO

With a pair of secateurs or a sharp knife, cut off a 5–10cm piece of stem and dip the cut end into hormone rooting powder, if using. Fill a small pot with suitable compost, insert the length of stem and water (you can put several cuttings into one pot). Cover with a plastic bag tied loosely around the base of the pot. If you are propagating an *Aeonium*, detach a rosette with about 5–10cm of stem attached and place the section of stem on its side. Leave for a few days to allow the base to heal over. Fill a small pot with cactus compost and gently insert the stem, firming around it to stabilise the plant, then water very sparingly. Do not cover.

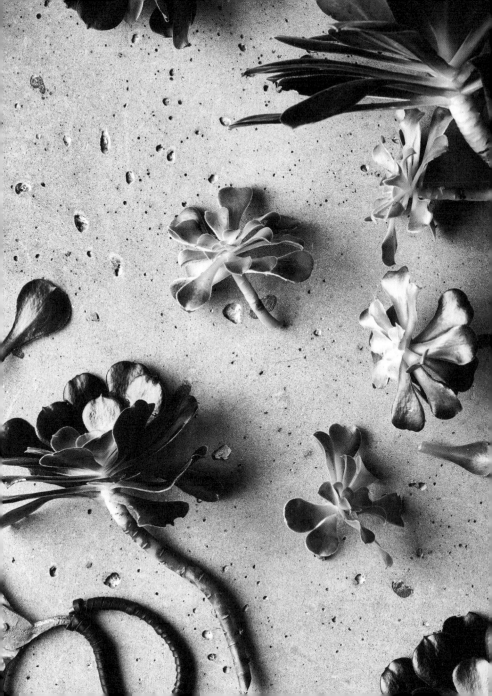

4 STEM CUTTINGS
IN WATER

+ CARE Keep the compost moist (but not wet) until new leaves form and grow the cutting on in a bright area out of direct sunlight.

SUITABLE PLANTS

Begonia
Heart Leaf Plant
Inch Plant (opposite)
Ivy
Mistletoe Cactus

Rooting plants in water is probably the easiest of all methods of propagation. Choose pretty glass vessels and line them up on a shelf to make a temporary display while waiting for your cuttings to sprout roots. For best results take cuttings 10–12cm in length during spring and summer, when they are usually more viable.

HOW TO

Cut off a 5cm length of stem, remove the lower leaves and place the cutting in a bottle or narrow-stemmed vase of water, choosing one that is just big enough to prop the stem up. The stem of the cutting naturally produces a hormone to encourage root growth from the stem buds. If the vessel you use is too large, the hormone will be more dilute in the water and the whole process of root growth will take longer. Roots should appear within a few weeks, but remember to refresh the water if it starts to look murky. When the roots are several centimetres long, remove the cutting and insert into a small pot of multi-purpose compost.

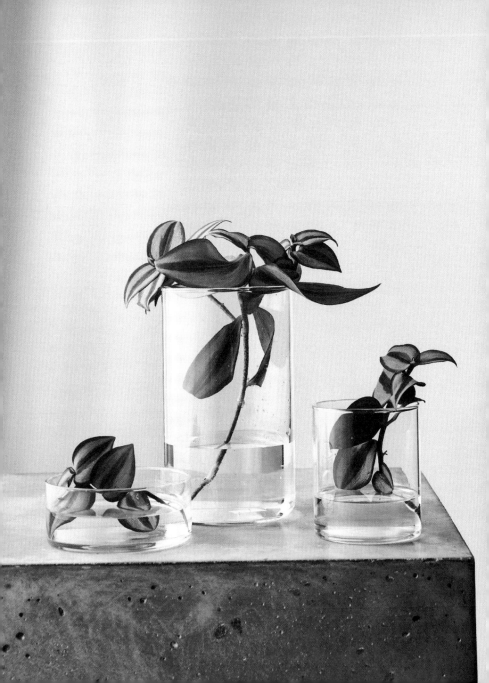

5 LEAF CUTTINGS

+ **CARE** Place the tray or pots in a bright, dry spot out of direct sunlight. Mist the leaves only very occasionally while waiting for the roots to develop.

SUITABLE PLANTS

Begonias
Cacti
Echeveria
Jade Plant
Panda Plant (opposite)
Snake Plant
and many succulents
and cacti

Although it seems unlikely that plants will grow roots from a single leaf, many do just that – especially succulents and cacti. You may even have noticed that a fallen leaf from an *Echeveria* will sprout if left on the surface of the compost.

HOW TO

Remove leaves from the parent plant using your thumb and forefinger to hold the leaf at the base where it connects with the stem. Firmly but gently twist until the whole leaf comes loose from the stem (the young plant will root from its base). You can also use leaves that have fallen naturally from the parent plant. Place the leaves in a dry place out of direct sunlight for a few days so the base can callous over, which is vital for new root growth. Fill a shallow tray or small pots with gritty compost and use a spray bottle to mist the surface, making sure not to over-moisten the compost, which will cause leaf rot. Simply lay the leaves of *Echeveria* on the surface of the compost where they will send out tiny roots. For other plants, especially cacti and succulents, insert the cut-end of the leaf into the compost to a depth of about 2cm. Within a few weeks you should notice new growth appearing.

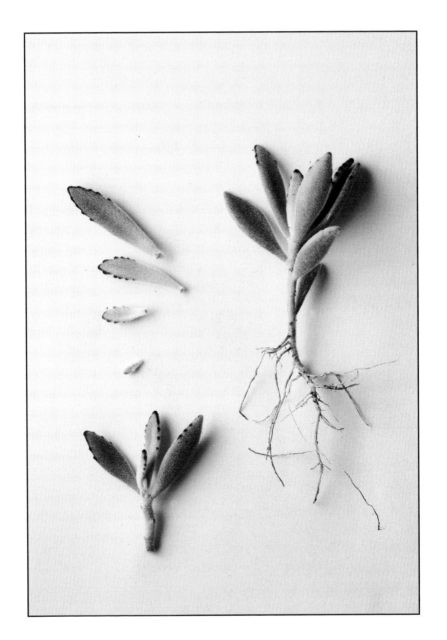

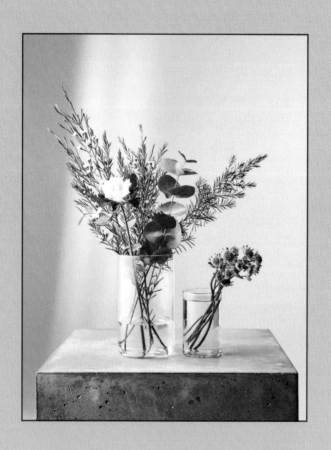

A plant

for

every

<u>room</u>

PLANTS

Air Plants
Kokedama Fern
Rubber Plant
String of Pearls
Urn Plant

PLANTS FOR A BATHROOM OR KITCHEN WITH NATURAL LIGHT

Most leafy plants love humidity and are suited to this atmosphere, but not succulents and most cacti: they retain moisture and will rot in a damp environment.

PLANTS

Boston Fern
Fishbone Cactus
Moth Orchid
Mikado African Spear
Spider Plant

PLANTS FOR A BATHROOM WITH LOW LIGHT

Many of us have bathrooms with just one small window, often with frosted glass that allows limited natural light to filter through. Fortunately, there are a number of humidity-loving plants from shady rainforests that will enjoy the low light levels.

PLANTS

Asparagus Fern
Chinese Evergreen
Parlour Palm
Peace Lily
Pin-stripe and other *Calathea* varieties
Polkadot Begonia

PLANTS FOR A SHADY CORNER

If you live in a basement flat or have a large room with limited natural light that doesn't reach the back or sides of the room, you may have given up hope of finding a suitable plant. But some houseplants can thrive in these conditions, preferring a spot away from bright, direct light.

PLANTS

Cacti (most)
Echeveria all varieties
Jade Plant
Ponytail Plant
Snake Plant

PLANTS FOR A SUNNY WINDOW SILL

A south-facing window sill is the perfect environment for sun-loving plants. But such bright, hot conditions don't suit leafier kinds so move them away from the window in the summer months.

PLANTS

Foxtail Fern
Heart Leaf
Inch Plant
Mistletoe Cactus
Staghorn Fern
String of Hearts

PLANTS FOR A MANTELPIECE OR SHELF

As long as there is sufficient natural light, this is the perfect spot for a range of trailing plants with attractive foliage that will cascade down. Choose a heavy pot to stabilise the plant and stop it from tipping forwards.

PLANTS

Bird's Nest Fern
Cast Iron Plant
Common or English Ivy
Cretan Brake Fern
Pothos Vine

PLANTS FOR A DRAUGHTY HALLWAY

Cold draughts and low light are not ideal conditions for tropical houseplants. But if you are determined to bring some life to a dingy hallway, a few tough plants out there will do the job.

PLANTS

African Spear
Cast Iron Plant
Echeveria
Kentia Palm
String of Pearls
Zebra Aloe

PLANTS FOR THE OFFICE

Modern offices often lack fresh air. Plants clean the air and create a much healthier space in which to work. When space is limited, go for plants that can sit on your desk or hang from a shelf.

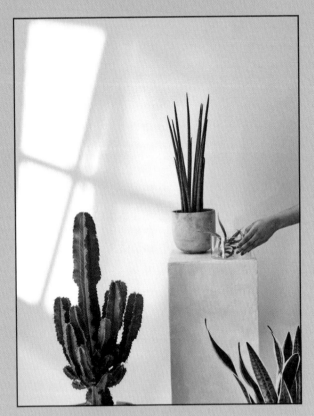

COWBOY CACTUS, 'MIKADO' AFRICAN SPEAR,
AIR PLANT AND SNAKE PLANT

CHAPTER 15

Ten

easy-going

plants

Whatever the conditions in your home and however inexperienced you are at growing things, the right plant for you is out there. And if you have a track record of killing plants, the cause is more likely to be too much care rather than too little. Overwatering, particularly in the winter months, is the number one killer of plants. If you have neglected your plant, don't be tempted to compensate by drowning it or giving it too much feed: you will literally be depriving the roots of oxygen and killing the plant with kindness. Always wait until the surface compost of the plant has dried out before re-wetting and you shouldn't go too far wrong. Here are my top ten starter plants. All are very robust and given just a little care and attention they will reward you amply.

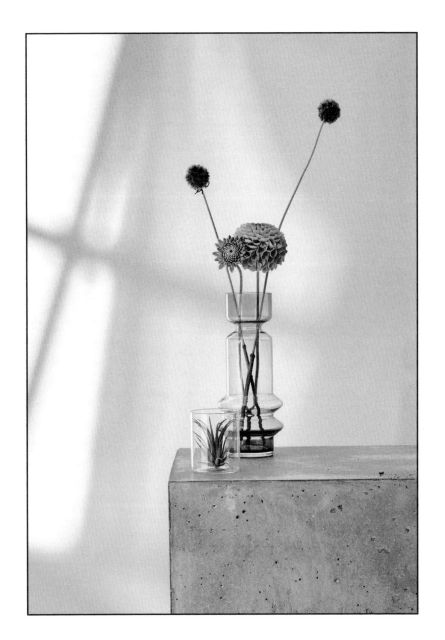

TEN EASY-GOING PLANTS

ALOE
ALOE VERA

Keep this plant in a sunny spot, but out of bright sunlight in the summer months. In the winter, the Aloe's fleshy, succulent leaves cope really well with the drying effect of central heating. Just make sure to water very sparingly and this healing plant will reward you with many offshoots, which can be potted on and shared with friends or used at home for cosmetics and juicing.

BIRD'S NEST FERN
ASPLENIUM NIDUS

There are so many great-looking ferns to choose from, but some varieties can be quite tricky to care for. Not this one, which is as tough as old boots. Preferring a cool spot out of bright sunlight, its luminous green leaves will light up a dingy corner.

CACTI

Try to replicate the dry, hot and sunny conditions that these desert-dwellers love and you won't go far wrong. Cacti are great plants for beginners – they store water so have few care needs but must never get their feet wet. Make sure they are in a pot with holes and that the compost is free draining. Symbolic of endurance and strength, these plants can cope with the most extreme conditions.

STRING OF HEARTS
CEROPEGIA WOODII

This most delicate of vines has adapted to cope with periods of drought by developing tubers near its roots. The tubers store water like mini-tanks, so the plant will cope with a great deal of neglect. Sit it up high on a shelf in bright, indirect light and marvel at just how fast this little plant grows in the summer. When the stems get too long they can be trimmed back and this will encourage bushier growth.

JADE PLANT
CRASSULA OVATA

Renowned for being virtually indestructible, this very dependable plant holds water in its stems and leaves and can tolerate dry conditions.

06

FISHBONE CACTUS
EPIPHYLLUM ANGULIGER

This rainforest plant from Central America grows high up in the canopy but out of bright sunlight, which would scorch its leaves. Other than indirect light, its only requirement is moderate watering. A good soak every couple of weeks should be sufficient for this easy-care but relatively uncommon plant. If you see one, snap it up and it may reward you with stunning scented flowers in summer.

HEART LEAF
PHILODENDRON SCANDENS

A beautiful, easy-going plant, this vine can tolerate low light levels and is very fast growing. It is perfect for training up walls on the shaded side of the room or cascading over the bannisters in a shady stairwell.

SNAKE PLANT
SANSEVIERIA

Very long-lived and pretty much indestructible, this plant will be with you for life. It is also known as the rough and tough plant, tolerating either low light or bright sun, so can handle whatever you throw at it. Just make sure not to overwater the compost or, eventually, the stems will rot.

09

UMBRELLA PLANT
SCHEFFLERA ARBORICOLA

Popular not only for its pretty palmate leaves but also on account of its tolerance of poor growing conditions, the Umbrella Plant copes with erratic watering as well as dry, centrally heated rooms. However, the plant will appreciate a good soak when the compost feels dry but make sure the pot has good drainage. If the plant sits in water the leaves will turn yellow and drop.

YUCCA

These large, statement plants can be quite an investment so choose a sturdy, good-looking plant that will go the distance. Yuccas are tough, love to bask in full sun and are quite drought tolerant. Choose a bright sunny spot for your plant, then water and feed freely throughout the summer months but make sure the compost never gets waterlogged. Your plant will quickly increase in size but if it outgrows its space, just cut the trunk back to the desired height. Leaves will soon sprout from the shortened stem.

RESOURCES

@BOTANYGEEK
Click on the igtv tab for informative planting guides.

@CLEVERBLOOM & WWW.CLEVERBLOOM.COM
Tips for beginner gardeners.

@HAARKON_ & WWW.HAARKON.CO.UK
Intriguing and calming global green adventures to flick through.

@JAMIES_JUNGLE
A London home with an awe-inspiring collection of tropical plants. A must follow for plant profiles and care too.

@LA_SIDHU
A UK-based plant fanatic with interiors to die for.

@LITTLEGREENFINGERS & WWW.LITTLEGREENFINGERS.DK
Living with plants in the smallest of flats.

@MUDDY_MADDIE
Qualified with the RHS, Maddie leads you into a world of botanical curiosities.

@NOUGHTICULTURE
Inspiration and advice on everything from propagation to reviving dying plants.

@SEEDTOSTEM & WWW.SEEDTOSTEMHOME.COM
Terrarium and biosphere inspiration.

@VERDUROUSWOMEN
Two women based in Portland showcase their amazing plants.

STOCKISTS

BOTANY
Beautifully curated store combining
homewares with houseplants.

CONSERVATORY ARCHIVES
For plant installations and plant hire.

FOREST
For hanging plants, leafy tropical plants and pots.

LONDON TERRARIUMS
Terrarium-making workshops and all the kit
to make your own terrariums.

N1 GARDEN CENTRE
For unusual and large specimen plants.

PRICK
For cacti and succulents.

EUROPE

LEAF, PARIS
A plant concept store selling ceramics from
artists and potters throughout France.

STALKS & ROOTS, COPENHAGEN
Huge flower shop with a large selection
of high-quality houseplants.

WILDERNIS, AMSTERDAM
An oasis of green in the centre of the city.

ZETA'S, STOCKHOLM
Indoor and outdoor plants set in a
beautiful garden.

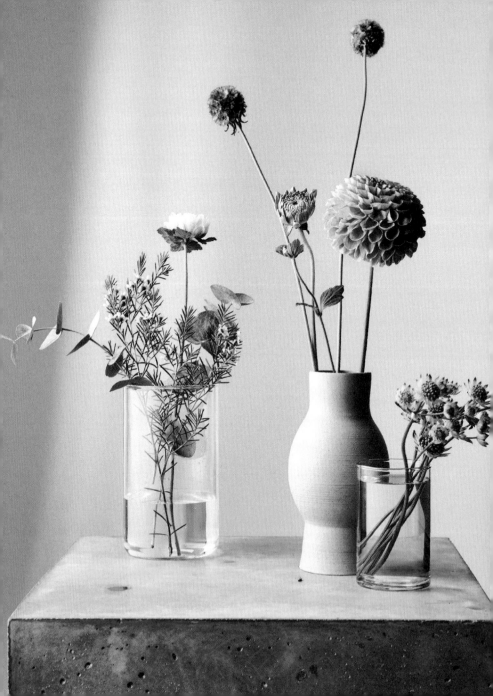

ABOUT
THE AUTHOR

Award-winning horticulturist Fran Bailey grew up on a cut flower nursery near York, where her Dutch father encouraged her love of all things botanical. After studying at the Welsh College of Horticulture she moved to London working as a freelance florist. Later she opened her first shop the Fresh Flower Company in South London expanding into houseplants with the opening of Forest in 2013, which she runs with the help of her daughters. Fran has written two other house plant books in collaboration with the RHS. Visit forest. london or follow @forest_london on Instagram.

THANKS

Fran Bailey would like to thank the team at Forest and Fresh Flower (in particular her daughters Alice, Maddie and Thea) for keeping the ship afloat in her absence.

Thank you to Elen Jones at Ebury Press for your encouragement and support, and to Caroline McArthur and Anna Kruger at whitefox. Finally, to Lucy at Imagist and Stephanie McLeod, whose beautiful plant portraits bring the book to life.

6

Pop Press, an imprint of
Ebury Publishing,

20 Vauxhall Bridge Road,
London SW1V 2SA

Pop Press is part of the
Penguin Random House
group of companies whose
addresses can be found at
global.penguinrandom
house.com

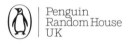

TEXT © Fran Bailey 2019

PHOTOGRAPHY
© Stephanie McLeod 2019

DESIGN BY Imagist

PROJECT MANAGEMENT BY whitefox

FIRST PUBLISHED BY
Pop Press in 2019

www.penguin.co.uk

A CIP catalogue record for this book is
available from the British Library

ISBN 9 7 8 1 5 2 9 1 0 4 0 6 6

COLOUR ORIGINATION BY Born

PRINTED AND BOUND in China
by Toppan Leefung

Penguin Random House is committed to a
sustainable future for our business, our readers
and our planet. This book is made from Forest
Stewardship Council® certified paper.

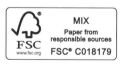